GROUP
PSYCHOTHERAPY
FOR WOMEN WITH
BREAST CANCER

GROUP PSYCHOTHERAPY
FOR WOMEN WITH
BREAST CANCER

James L. Spira, PhD, MPH, ABPP,
and Geoffrey M. Reed, PhD

American Psychological Association
Washington, DC

Published by
American Psychological Association
750 First Street, NE
Washington, DC 20002
www.apa.org

To order
APA Order Department
P.O. Box 92984
Washington, DC 20090-2984
Tel: (800) 374-2721; Direct: (202) 336-5510
Fax: (202) 336-5502; TDD/TTY: (202) 336-6123
Online: www.apa.org/books/
Email: order@apa.org

In the U.K., Europe, Africa, and the Middle East, copies may be ordered from
American Psychological Association
3 Henrietta Street
Covent Garden, London
WC2E 8LU England

Typeset in Meridien by EPS Group Inc., Easton, MD

Printer: Automated Graphic Systems, White Plains, MD
Cover Designer: Naylor Design, Washington, DC
Technical/Production Editor: Casey Ann Reever

The opinions and statements published are the responsibility of the authors, and such opinions and statements do not necessarily represent the policies of the American Psychological Association.

Library of Congress Cataloging-in-Publication Data
Spira, James L.
  Group psychotherapy for women with breast cancer : a treatment manual / James L. Spira and Geoffrey M. Reed.
       p. cm.
     Includes bibliographical references and index.
     ISBN 1-55798-955-9 (alk. paper)
       1. Breast—Cancer—Patients—Mental health.   2. Group psychotherapy.
   I. Reed, Geoffrey M.   II. Title.
   RC280.B8 S5895 2002
   616.99'449'0019—dc21

                                                                            2002008093

British Library Cataloguing-in-Publication Data
A CIP record is available from the British Library.

Printed in the United States of America
First Edition

Contents

Acknowledgments

This project began in 1996 as a treatment manual developed for a research project jointly conducted by the American Psychological Association (APA) and Blue Cross/Blue Shield of Massachusetts. From its inception, this project was conceived and supported by the APA Practice Directorate. We are grateful to Russ Newman, PhD, JD, Executive Director for Professional Practice at APA, for the vision and insight that made this book possible. Over the course of the project we received considerable support and input for the manual from a variety of people associated with the project, including Ava Stanton; LCSW, Janet Bailey, EdD; Stan Berman, PhD; Marc Schulz, PhD; Laura Basili, PhD; Gerry Koocher, PhD; and Sandy Haber, PhD. Thanks also to Lansing Hays and Vanessa Downing for their editing of the manuscript.

Influences on this approach to therapy come from many personal mentors. Foremost among them is Irvin Yalom, MD, who first conducted group psychotherapy with a group of breast cancer patients 25 years ago and whose seminal influence on the current research and clinical popularity of group therapy for women with breast cancer is without comparison. But it is without a doubt the women in the groups themselves who have been the principal teachers and major developers of this manual. Their struggles, insights, and lessons have both inspired and informed what follows.

GROUP PSYCHOTHERAPY

FOR WOMEN WITH

BREAST CANCER

An Introduction to the Treatment Model

1

This book is intended to provide a clinical framework for health professionals who wish to offer group psychosocial support to breast cancer patients. The model described here is most specifically designed to help women with a first occurrence of breast cancer. However, this approach can easily be adapted to breast cancer patients at other stages of disease and to other populations, and this book provides guidance for other applications. On its own, this book is intended primarily for experienced group therapists. We hope that it will also be a useful part of a broader set of training resources for those new to the field. Whereas researchers may find this book useful as a manual for training therapists as part of specific research protocols, our primary purpose for this book is to guide clinicians who wish to provide group therapy for women with breast cancer in actual clinical settings.

This book is based on thousands of hours spent conducting group therapy over the past 20 years and more than 10 years of experience with developing and using treatment manuals for breast cancer and other chronically ill patients and training therapists in their use. The treatment model described in this book is partly based on a treatment approach developed by Irvin Yalom and his colleagues at Stanford University (see Spiegel, Bloom, & Yalom, 1981). However, it also incorporates a variety of other methods and theoretical traditions. An earlier version of this manual was developed for the implementation of a research project intended to demonstrate whether group psychotherapy for breast cancer patients could be effectively integrated into a community setting and whether it could improve the quality of life and physical health of breast cancer patients (Spiegel & Spira, 1991). This approach was further modified and elaborated as part of a project conducted by the American Psychological Association Practice Directorate to integrate psychosocial care into the treatment of women with breast cancer in a large health care system (Spira & Reed, 1996). This book incorporates significant refinements, additions, and modifications of these early efforts.

The model of group psychotherapy described here can be implemented by a variety of health care professionals (e.g., psychologists, social workers, nurses) in a variety of settings. Group therapy can be conducted in a private practice or small clinic setting, and it can also be readily integrated into a large medical setting in a collaborative effort with medical personnel to improve the psychological well-being of breast cancer patients. We have found that this manual can be used by

- clinicians who want to help patients improve their quality of life,
- researchers who want a manual-guided intervention to examine the efficacy of psychosocial intervention for quality-of-life or health outcomes, and
- health care providers who want a better understanding of the psychosocial factors associated with living with and recovering from breast cancer.

Why Group Psychotherapy?

Group therapy specifically designed for people with medical illness is one of the most powerful forms of intervention available to them. Although individual treatment can certainly be useful in a variety of settings, group therapy offers several unique benefits. In what is generally considered the authoritative work on group therapy, Yalom (1985) described several curative factors in the group setting that contribute to patient improvement. First among these is universality—the opportunity for group members to feel that they are not alone in their situation. Being part of a group offers a sense of community that diminishes feelings of alienation and isolation that may be particularly acute for patients with life-threatening illness. The second is altruism, which gives group members a sense of purpose. Through lending support and guidance to others in the group, one's own life is given an additional sense of meaning. The third is perhaps the most important for breast cancer patients: hope. Group members have an opportunity to see that others experience the same emotions and cope with similar—or even worse—circumstances as themselves. Yet, others are also able to experience meaning in life and often a good quality of life. This instills hope that they, too, can handle these situations. Because of the power of these shared experiences, a group format is especially beneficial to medically ill patients (Spira, 1997b).

Group therapy should never replace individual treatment when individual treatment is indicated. For those patients who are appropriate candidates for group treatment, however, group therapy is often more cost-effective than individual treatment (Benezra, 1990). Group psychotherapy may be up to four times more affordable for patients and equally as cost-effective for health care organizations (Yalom & Yalom, 1990). This may be particularly relevant in the treatment of medical populations who are undergoing a variety of medical procedures and who may be paying out of pocket for expensive complementary treatments.

Using This Manual for Therapist Training

We hope that this book provides a valuable introduction for those with less clinical experience. However, this book alone is clearly insufficient as a training tool for individuals without other experience with psychotherapy. We believe that this manual will be used most effectively by licensed psychotherapists

- who work with cancer patients but may lack group therapy experience,
- who have other group experience and wish to begin treating cancer patients, and
- who already work with breast cancer groups but are interested in some fresh ideas.

Under these circumstances, the manual should help sensitize therapists to aspects of group psychotherapy for breast cancer patients they might not have previously considered and facilitate their training and supervision in this area. However, as with any new psychotherapy skill, appropriate supervision by an experienced teacher or colleague is mandatory.

Psychotherapy for cancer groups requires a wide range of therapeutic skills, considerable life experience, and a certain maturity for dealing with essential life and life-threatening issues. A single therapist experienced in leading cancer groups can effectively implement this intervention. However, it is difficult to find all the requisite skills in a single individual. For this reason, cotherapists with complementary skills form an ideal team for implementing this model. In deciding who should facilitate these groups, a range of qualities and skills shared between therapists should be considered. Additional information about the cotherapy model is presented in chapter 4.

Goals and Methods of Intervention

In brief, the goals of the intervention are to help group members adjust to the diagnosis of the breast cancer, to cope with the sequelae of cancer treatment, and to adjust to living with breast cancer by considering the impact and meaning of the cancer in their lives. On the basis of the literature and our clinical experience, we have developed an intervention with two major components to facilitate coping and adjustment: a psychotherapeutic component and a self-guided psychoeducational component. The treatment approach we describe uses both this book for therapists and a companion, *The Breast Cancer Notebook: The Healing Power of Reflection* (Stanton & Reed, 2002) for patients (see Exhibit 1.1).

THE PSYCHOEDUCATIONAL COMPONENT

The psychoeducational materials developed for this group are published as a separate volume, *The Breast Cancer Notebook: The Healing Power of Reflection* (Stanton & Reed, 2002). Meant to complement the psychotherapeutic sessions, *The Breast Cancer Notebook* is ideally given to patients before the first group session (following a pregroup intake interview; see chapter 4). The notebook contains materials meant to assist group members in exploring many of the issues that commonly arise over the course of the 16-week group psychotherapy. It is divided into 12 chapters or topic areas. Group members are encouraged to read and answer the questions that they find relevant to their individual concerns or that the group

---

EXHIBIT 1.1

Comparison of the Psychotherapeutic and Psychoeducational Components

Psychotherapeutic Component *Group Psychotherapy for Women With Breast Cancer*		Psychoeducational Component *The Breast Cancer Notebook*
For therapists		For group members
Offers general principles and specific techniques to facilitate group process	↔	Information and self-review questions to stimulate group members' exploration of issues
For use in group meetings		For use between meetings

may be currently exploring. Their experiences with the notebook often serve to stimulate discussion of relevant issues they wish to bring up in the next weekly group discussion. A particular topic can be pursued in more depth by referring to other books and resources listed.

The Breast Cancer Notebook is intended to correspond to the expected progress of the group. In the beginning sessions, specific exercises are assigned that relate thematically to the topics expected to be initially raised in the group meetings. Integration of the notebook during later sessions should begin to occur more naturally through questions and reactions that members bring back to the group after reviewing the material or by being directed to aspects of the notebook that correspond to issues they raised in the group that week. More specific information about integrating *The Breast Cancer Notebook* with the group therapy is presented in chapters 4 and 7.

We have found that the method presented here of augmenting the group sessions with separately presented educational information and opportunities for self-guided exploration of themes does two things: (a) It keeps the group sessions focused on the supportive and expressive elements of therapy that are unique to the group context (and correspondingly free of the tendency to focus on "information"), and (b) it allows continuity of support throughout the week by encouraging patients to become more active through journaling and self-guided exercises.

Patients with a first occurrence of breast cancer will probably find most of these issues of relevance to them, depending on the time since their diagnosis. Patients with recurrent breast cancer will probably find many of these topics to be still relevant, although their perspective may have undergone a change because they previously dealt with many of these issues during their initial diagnosis and treatment.

THE PSYCHOTHERAPEUTIC COMPONENT

The psychotherapeutic component is the primary focus of this manual. In brief, the therapeutic approach is intended to assist group members to reduce distress and to live as fully and authentically as possible in each moment of their lives by doing the following:

- openly and calmly addressing any issue related to living with breast cancer and the impact of this experience on participants' lives;
- expressing freely with open affect, without avoidance of negative thoughts or feelings;
- drawing on the emotional support and understanding of others;
- finding ways to become actively involved with the difficulties one is facing; and
- using the crisis as an opportunity for growth.

Toward this end, therapists allow group members to discuss any concern that is relevant for them in the group, and they focus the intervention on the quality of group members' expression during the therapeutic sessions rather than focusing on any particular topic. By demonstrating rapport and asking leading questions, therapists encourage group members to discuss their concerns in personal and concrete terms, with open affect; to interact with each other as much as possible; and to search for ways to actively participate in areas they otherwise feel reluctant to explore. Emphasis is placed on examining underlying assumptions about their lives, reflecting on those that limit as well as those that enhance meaning and purpose. Every opportunity is given to re-evaluate priorities so that group members are able to adjust to current circumstances, thus allowing them to live as fully as possible in each moment and in full relationship with those they care about. The therapeutic strategies used to achieve these ends are explored in more detail throughout this manual (see Exhibit 1.2).

The methods of group psychotherapy described here are influenced by several complementary psychotherapeutic methods, including classical cognitive, interpersonal, and existential approaches. They are also strongly influenced by basic counseling methods and the group work of Irvin Yalom (1985).

This approach is also guided by research on psychosocial factors influencing quality of life and physical health of cancer patients. Chapter 2 reviews some of this relevant literature.

EXHIBIT 1.2

Author's Assumption Regarding Health and Distress

In brief, the approach delineated in this manual assumes that optimal health occurs when she is able to

- spend the majority of one's time focused on the moment,
- have a sense of well-being, at least for part of each day,
- openly and honestly express and receive thoughts and feelings with those she cares about, and
- daily have the opportunity to regularly engage in an activity that is full of meaning, purpose, and value.

We consider one to be in a distressed state when one

- is distracted by past or future worries a majority of one's time;
- experiences constant pain, stress, or anhedonia;
- is unable to recognize, express, or act on one's thoughts and feelings;
- lacks the opportunity to regularly engage in meaningful, purposeful, and valuable activities.

Psychosocial Factors and Interventions Affecting Patient Outcomes

2

This chapter provides an overview of some of the current scientific evidence that provides a foundation for the intervention approach recommended in this book. This literature relates to problems encountered by cancer patients, particularly breast cancer patients, including psychosocial adjustment, daily functioning, and treatment compliance. Here we discuss the potential effectiveness of psychosocial interventions in addressing quality-of-life issues, and we briefly review the literature suggesting the potential benefits of psychosocial interventions on immunological and health outcomes. We also address the recent controversy regarding the effect of breast cancer support groups on survival. We believe that it is important for group therapists to be generally familiar with this literature, although it is not as directly useful for training purposes as the material in the chapters that follow.

Rather than presenting a comprehensive literature review, we provide an overview of the research base that guides our intervention approach. Readers interested in a more complete review of the research related to psychosocial interventions for cancer are referred to Baum and Anderson (2001); to Spira (1997b) for a description of group interventions with other medical populations; and to Haber (1995) for a broader clinical description of the psychological treatment of breast cancer patients.

Do Psychological Factors Affect the Course of Cancer?

Whereas there is little evidence that psychological factors cause cancer, several human studies have found associations between coping patterns or other responses to cancer and cancer outcomes such as recurrence and mortality (e.g., Derogatis, Abeloff, & Melisaratos, 1979; Levy, Lee, Bagley, & Lippman, 1988; Rogentine et al., 1979; Watson & Greer, 1998). Other studies, however, have found no such relationships (e.g., Cassileth, Lusk, Miller, Brown, & Miller, 1985; Jamison, Burish, & Wallston, 1987; Zonderman, Costa, & McCrae, 1989). Many of these studies are limited by their failure to control longitudinally for potentially confounding biological, psychological, and behavioral variables. At this point, no definitive conclusion can be drawn.

One unfortunate by-product of the interest in this area has been that sometimes breast cancer patients feel that the "wrong" emotional response to cancer may place them somehow at greater risk. The approach we describe in this book assumes that the authentic expression of group members' emotional responses in a way that they can control and within a supportive context provides the most benefit to their adjustment over time. That is, there are no wrong responses.

Another frequent question relates to the role of stress in cancer. A number of studies have suggested that uncontrollable stress can increase the rate of tumor metastases in animals (e.g., Ben-Eliyahu, Yirmiya, Liebeskind, Taylor, & Gale, 1991; see Herberman, 1991, for a review). However, similar studies have not been conducted with human participants for obvious reasons. Behavioral factors that may be associated with stress, such as smoking, lack of exercise, use of alcohol and other substances, and poor nutrition, are also contributors to poor health outcomes. The treatment approach described in this book assumes that teaching group members techniques to manage and reduce stress enhances the quality of their lives, regardless of its potential impact on the course of their disease. This intervention, through the *The Breast Cancer Notebook: The Healing Power of Reflection* (Stanton & Reed, 2002), also incorporates information regarding the importance of positive health behaviors.

How Difficult Is It to Adjust to Cancer?

A diagnosis of cancer may be among the most profound stressors a person can face. Individuals diagnosed with cancer often face uncertainties about the length of life available to them, the future course of their illness, their ability to care for themselves, their present and future physical capacities, and the experience of symptoms. Empirical studies have documented severe emotional distress in response to the diagnosis (e.g., Andersen, Anderson, & deProsse, 1989) as well as chronic stress reactions as a function of lengthy cancer treatments and disruptions in major life areas (e.g., Cella & Tross, 1986; see Andersen, Kiecolt-Glaser, & Glaser, 1994, for a review). Chronic stressors experienced by cancer patients may include disrupted life tasks, social and interpersonal turmoil, fatigue and low energy, sexual problems, disturbances in intimate relationships and social support, unemployment or underemployment, job discrimination, and difficulties in obtaining health insurance. All of these stressors may contribute significantly to emotional distress. Estimates of the prevalence of depressive symptoms in cancer patients range from 20% to 58% (Craig & Abeloff, 1974; Plumb & Holland, 1977). More recently, research has noted the prevalence rates of a psychiatric disorder to be 45%, with a prevalence rate of 42% of anxiety and depressive diagnoses (Kissane et al., 1998). Rates of posttraumatic stress symptoms are also elevated among cancer patients (Cordova et al., 1995).

Behavioral symptoms related to psychological stress from cancer include appetite disturbances manifested by eating less often and eating meals of lower nutritional value, often unrelated to problems such as nausea and vomiting (e.g., Wellisch, Wolcott, Pasnau, Fawzy, & Landsverk, 1989). Chronic sleep problems are also reported by a significant proportion of cancer patients (e.g., Cella & Tross, 1986). Individuals experiencing psychological stress or distress are also more likely to self-medicate with alcohol or other drugs (Grunberg & Baum, 1985) or to increase cigarette smoking or caffeine consumption. Poor health behaviors may potentiate the effects of stress, and their occurrence with cancer may add psychological and biological burdens. Cancer stressors may also decrease the frequency of positive health behaviors such as physical exercise, which may have benefits in terms of both mood and functional capacity (see Andersen et al., 1994, for a review).

Breast cancer treatments such as chemotherapy and radiation can have such serious physical and psychological side effects that it is often difficult for cancer patients to comply with recommended treatments. Noncompliance with treatment, in turn, may decrease the effectiveness of medical care and even adversely affect survival. Ayres and colleagues (1994) found that 37% of breast cancer patients kept less than 85% of their clinic appointments for intravenous-administered chemotherapy, and noncompliance with oral chemotherapy may be even higher. Depressive and other psychological symptoms are thought to be related to noncompliance (Ayers et al., 1994; Richardson et al., 1987; Richardson, Marks, & Levine, 1988). In some cases, psychological difficulties associated with breast cancer may be so disruptive that patients become discouraged and stop treatment altogether (see Andersen et al., 1994).

How Can Group Interventions Help?

Psychosocial intervention programs, particularly those offered in a group format, have been shown to substantially reduce the emotional distress associated with cancer, provide important social support, and enhance adaptive coping skills (e.g., Ali & Khalil, 1989; Cain, Kohorn, Quinlan, Latimer, & Schwartz, 1986; Cunningham, 1989; Fawzy, Cousins, et al., 1990; Forester, Kornfeld, Fleiss, & Thompson, 1993; Heinreich & Schag, 1985; Johnson, 1982; Spiegel et al., 1981; Telch & Telch, 1986; see Baum & Anderson, 2001, for comprehensive reviews). These findings have been consistent in studies over the past 30 years. However, some recent studies have suggested that the benefits of these group interventions may not be sustained over time (e.g., Edmonds, Lockwood, & Cummingham, 1999; Edelman, Bell, & Kidman, 1999). Therefore, the treatment model described in this book focuses partly on developing skills in group members that are more likely to be sustained for longer periods of time.

In addition, a variety of studies have focused on the benefits of psychoeducational programs, often offered in a group format. In their meta-analysis of 116 studies, Devine and Westlake (1995) have found that psychoeducational approaches tended to achieve significant decreases in pain, nausea, and vomiting. Helgeson, Cohen, Schulz, and Yasko (1999) found that an education-based group intervention improved initial adjustment to a diagnosis of breast cancer as compared to a peer discussion group. These approaches can also help to improve communication between patients and their health care providers, which in turn has been demonstrated to improve patients' understanding of their disease and treatment, their retention of medical information, their satisfaction with health care, and their compliance with treatment (see Andersen et al., 1994). Side effects may be better tolerated, and more effective communication about the patient's experiences may help to minimize them. Aspects of the intervention model described in this book therefore focus on providing relevant educational materials, particularly through the use of *The Breast Cancer Notebook*, and providing opportunities to discuss these materials in the group.

Experiential methods are also showing promise in helping breast cancer patients to improve their quality of life and possibly their physical health. Kabat-Zinn's group at the University of Massachusetts (Massion, Teas, Hebert, Wertheimer, & Kabat-Zinn, 1995) found that Buddhism-style meditation improved breast and prostate patients' quality of life and also increased melatonin levels. Hypnosis has also been found to improve cancer patients' ability to cope with treatment as well as boost overall quality of life (Spira & Spiegel, 1992; Steggles, Maxwell, Lightfoot, Damore-Petingola, & Mayer, 1997). Relaxation–biofeedback has long been known to enhance cancer patients' ability to reduce stress and tolerate chemotherapy (Morrow et al., 1999). Therapists who are familiar with these types of techniques can incorporate them into the model of intervention presented here during the periods of each group session that are devoted to relaxation.

Interest in group interventions as possible enhancers of cancer patients' immune functioning has been based on the idea that the progression of certain types of cancer may be partly mediated by the immune system. Fawzy, Fawzy, Hyun, and Wheeler (1997) found that patients with malignant melanoma who improved active cognitive and behavioral coping also showed improvements in several immune parameters. This type of research is difficult to evaluate, because cancer patients undergoing oncotherapy have very unstable immune systems, and the relationship between immune factors and health outcome is unclear. This area warrants further investigation, and multimillion dollar grants have been awarded to several research centers to try to overcome these difficulties. These results will not be available for some years.

Can Group Therapy Prolong Survival for Cancer Patients?

The effect of group therapy on prolonged survival has recently become an area of considerable interest and great controversy. Two intervention studies have suggested that group psychotherapy may affect the survival of cancer patients. Interested in determining the influence that Irvin Yalom's approach to group therapy for women with breast cancer might have on their health, David Spiegel, Joan Bloom, and other colleagues at Stanford University studied women with metastatic breast cancer who had poor prognoses. Intervention participants met weekly in psychological intervention groups for at least 1 year. The group approach was based on the work of Irvin Yalom (1980, 1985) and focused on the expression of emotional experience related to cancer in the context of group support (see Spiegel et al., 1981, and Spiegel & Spira, 1991, for a description). At 12-month follow-up, intervention participants exhibited less psychological distress, less depression, fewer maladaptive coping responses, and fewer phobias than did control participants (Spiegel et al., 1981). Moreover, at 10-year follow-up, survival times for intervention participants were approximately 18 months longer than control participants when calculated from the time they joined the study (Spiegel, Bloom, Kraemer, & Gottheil, 1989).

The second study that found a beneficial effect of intervention on survival involved a different cancer population. Fawzy and his colleagues at the University of California at Los Angeles conducted a 6-week structured group intervention for newly diagnosed malignant melanoma patients with good prognoses. The intervention consisted of health education, enhancement of problem-solving and coping skills regarding participants' disease, stress management and relaxation techniques, and psychological support. At 6-month follow-up, these researchers found significantly lower depression and improved mood, as well as more adaptive coping strategies among intervention participants as compared to control participants (Fawzy, Cousins, et al., 1990). Aspects of immune functioning were also improved among intervention participants (Fawzy, Kemeny, et al., 1990). In a later follow-up study, these researchers have reported a lower proportion of cancer recurrence and death among intervention participants as compared to controls over a 6-year follow-up period (Fawzy et al., 1993). Thirty-eight percent of patients who had not undergone the intervention had either had a recurrence of their cancer or had died, compared to only 21% of the intervention participants.

Of these two studies, the Spiegel study at Stanford has attracted more attention and more controversy. To date, attempts to replicate the findings of this study have not been successful. In 1990, Spiegel received a large National Institutes of Health grant to conduct a 5-year prospective randomized study to determine whether women with recurrent breast cancer can indeed extend survival through group psychotherapy. More than 12 years later, and with more than double the sample of the original study, Spiegel's group has yet to report survival benefits related to psychotherapy. However, they have reported improved quality of life in the treatment group (Classen et al., 2001). In a related multicenter trial conducted by Goodwin and colleagues (2001) throughout Canada, more than 200 women with recurrent breast cancer were treated in a similar fashion as in the Spiegel study (citing the Spiegel & Spira, 1991, training manual and receiving training from the Spiegel group). Once again, quality of life improved for the treatment group, but no survival benefits were found. Applauding the thoroughness of the Goodwin study and commenting on studies that purport to find survival benefits, Dr. Jimmie Holland, Chief of Psychiatry at Memorial Sloan–Kettering Cancer Center in New York, remarked, "Even if the study is flawed, like the [Spiegel et al., 1989] one that found that women in support groups survived longer, people may want to believe it because it's such an appealing idea" (p. 36; Holland, 2001). The Goodwin report went on to discuss the value of improved quality of life, despite the decreasing hope that survival can be prolonged.

Fox (1998) offered an epidemiological hypothesis about Spiegel's original finding and his inability to replicate the survival findings. He noted that because the control survival curve looked unusually steep, lacking an expected right-skewed tail, both the treatement and control mortality curves were compared (by Fox) with that of a population from the same region having metastatic breast cancer. When transformed to life table format, the curves of the control sample and the regional population (neither group having had an intervention) were almost identical for a year and then differed strikingly after 20 months. It appears that the control group (N = 36) died at a faster rate than would be expected. Whereas the treatment group in Spiegel's study lived no longer than would be expected when compared to the general population of metastatic breast cancer patients. Fox concluded that "the intervention had no effect; that the intervention curve was in fact equivalent to a control curve with mild sampling departure from that of the regional population; and that, therefore, the repetition of the study now under way would not yield confirmation of the 1989 study . . ." (p. 361). Nor has it to this date.

In another large multicenter trial examining the benefits of group short-term (16 weeks) psychotherapy on women with a first occurrence of breast cancer, Spiegel et al. (1999) also were unable to determine whether survival differences were attributable to intervention. However, this project (based on Spiegel & Spira, 1991, and in which Spira was involved in the training and evaluations of therapists) did demonstrate that the style of group therapy presented in this book can be learned by health professionals and implemented effectively, in terms of therapists adequately delivering the intervention and helping patients improve their quality of life.

Other researchers have also been unable to find an association between survival and various forms of group intervention, including a group treatment approach based on the work of Bernie Siegel (Gellert, Maxwell, & Siegel, 1993), emphasizing thoughts of a more positive future without dwelling on the negative. Studies by Cunningham et al. (1998) and Edelman et al. (1999) have not found a survival benefit of other group approaches. Yet, improvements in psychological functioning and quality of life are also noted in these studies.

Which Group Approach Is Best?

A meta-analysis was performed for of all prospective randomized studies examining the effects of educational, behavioral, and counseling interventions for cancer patients (Meyer & Mark, 1995). Not surprisingly, informational and educational approaches were most effective in improving medical knowledge and compliance as well as functional adjustment, behavioral approaches were most effective with managing specific symptoms, and nonbehavioral counseling therapy was superior for assisting with emotional adjustment as well as in more global measures examined. Also noteworthy is that support groups that lacked psychotherapeutic interventions were not found to be of value for any outcomes examined. In their 1995 study, Evans and Connis compared a cognitive–behavioral therapy (CBT) group with a social support group and a no treatment control group. Consistent with Meyer and Mark's review, Evans and Cannis found that CBT and social support were better than no treatment. Interestingly, they noted that the social support group was superior to the CBT group and resulted in lower psychiatric symptoms, lower maladaptive sensitivity, and lower anxiety. Additionally, they found that the social support group exhibited more changes at 6 months when compared with the CBT group and the no treatment group (Evans & Cannis, 1995). Most recently, Helgeson Cohen, Schulz, and Yasko (2000) at Carnegie–Mellon University have been conducting a series of studies to determine which forms of therapy are most effective for women with breast cancer. They have shown that for women with early-stage cancer who are coping better with their situation tend to prefer and respond better to psychoeducational approaches, whereas women with more advanced stages of cancer and with poorer social support benefit from more supportive psychotherapy. This new line of investigation, inquiring into which types of patients respond best to which types of therapy, is an important trend in psychosocial oncology and one that all clinical interventions should take into consideration.

A Final Note

Based on the literature review presented above, we present below a method of group psychotherapy for women with a first occurrence of breast cancer (with a longer option for women with recurrent breast cancer) that is 16 weeks in duration, emphasizes interpersonal psychotherapy with emotional and supportive elements (and supported by cognitive and existential therapy approaches), and which includes a separate psychoeducational component for women with first occurrence breast cancer. This approach also involves teaching experiential skills (relaxation, meditation, and self-hypnosis). The model allows therapists the flexibility to emphasize a more supportive or skills-based therapy to accommodate a wide range of patients' needs. Our experience has shown us that these approaches can be synthesized to offer a powerful treatment, one that benefits most patients.

It would be extremely unfortunate if the effect of the failure to confirm survival benefits as a result of group psychotherapy for cancer patients resulted in either a withdrawal of support for these programs by the institutions that have supported them or the perception that the groups are not of benefit. We cannot overstate our belief that improvements in quality of life and subjective quality of experience are more than sufficient justification for providing these services to women with breast cancer and to other patients. We believe that the availability of these services should be a standard part of medical care. We are also intimately aware of the tremendous meaning of these groups for many —if not most—of the women who have participated in the groups we have conducted. The richness of their experience and its personal significance simply cannot be adequately captured by standardized outcome measures. It is in this spirit that we offer this book.

Therapeutic Approach

3

Understanding how group therapy for cancer patients differs from both individual therapy and group psychotherapy for people with a psychosocial disturbance provides a foundation for understanding the power as well as the limitations of the protocol outlined in this book.

Group vs. Individual Treatment

Whereas group therapy has tremendous potential to assist most cancer patients, individual psychotherapy can be of incomparable value for certain individuals, especially those with a preexisting psychological disturbance or personality characteristics that make it difficult for them to cope with treatment and to adjust to living with cancer or precludes them from interacting successfully in a group setting (see Haber, 1995; Trijsburg, van Knippenberg, & Rijpma, 1992). Yet even many of these patients can be assisted by the approach to group therapy we describe here. Therefore, whenever possible, our approach to group therapy can be considered the "treatment of choice" for most cancer patients.

In contrast to the usual emphasis on examining and modifying personality patterns prevalent in individual therapy, group therapy for people with cancer emphasizes living more fully in each moment and garnering supportive experiences from others in coping with the stresses of life as a cancer patient. Certainly individual therapy can assist patients with such adjustments, and group therapy can assist in modifying personality patterns. However, each is better suited to different problems because of the context in which it operates. In individual therapy, the therapist can focus on the complex puzzle that comprises each person's life, whereas a group setting is better suited to use the invaluable experience of others in coping with and adjusting to issues common to most cancer patients. Nowhere can the power of the group be more beneficially used than with breast cancer patients.

Group psychotherapy for women with breast cancer has a natural foundation. These women have the following characteristics in common:

- their gender (generally more conducive to group discussion than men's groups),
- a disease that is life-threatening yet inconsistent in its course,
- a cancer site and corresponding treatments that affect the very heart of their femininity, and
- surprisingly common psychosocial concerns (see the discussion of typical themes in chapter 5).

These factors, together with minimal yet important therapist intervention, combine to induce strangers to form a coherent supportive milieu that can foster psychosocial and possibly health improvements.

Group Therapy for People With Psychosocial Disturbance vs. People With Cancer

Traditionally, group psychotherapy has been conducted for people with various psychosocial issues (Yalom, 1985), yet members are selected to participate on the basis of similar levels of ego functioning (homogenous cognitive functioning, heterogeneous presenting concern). A typical group focus is relationship difficulties that are variable in nature. Ever more popular today are general broad-based support groups, such as women's groups, men's groups, gay and lesbian support groups, groups for military enlisted personnel, and so on. These groups may or may not be led by a therapist, and they may comprise diverse individuals with an equally diverse range of issues, with only a thin thread of commonality (heterogeneous cognitive functioning, heterogeneous presenting concern). Other groups may focus on a particular diagnosis, such as major depressive disorder, anxiety disorder, or schizophrenia. Patients are selected to participate on the basis of their diagnosis and level of ego functioning (homogenous cognitive functioning, homogenous presenting concern).

Group therapy for people with a medical illness is very different from group therapy for people with a psychological illness, however. A serious illness can attack anyone at any time. Therefore, these groups typically consist of people with a wide range of past experiences, personal and external resources, and personality styles. Nonetheless, they may or usually have much in common. Typical themes discussed in groups of cancer patients include communication with medical professionals; relationships with family, friends, and coworkers; coping with medical treatment and effects of the disease; adjusting to living with a cancer diagnosis; and existential issues such as addressing the possibility of dying, examining one's priorities, and shifting self-image (Spira, 1991; Spira & Spiegel, 1993). Although cancer patients deal with many common issues, the range of personality types in these groups is as varied as may be found in the general population (heterogeneous cognitive functioning, homogenous presenting concern). In this way, groups with a psychosocial focus differ from those comprising medically ill individuals (see Table 3.1).

For people with interpersonal concerns, group therapy most typically follows an interpersonal format (Yalom, 1985). Group therapy for people with a psychological diagnosis typically uses a cognitive–behavioral therapy (CBT) approach (Beck, Rush, Shaw, & Emery, 1979) or a hybrid interpersonal therapy approach (Klerman, Weissman, Rounsavill, & Chevron, 1984). More general support groups use a psychoeducational structure possibly facilitated by a general counseling style (Carkhuff, 2000).

Group therapy for cancer patients includes a variety of formats, ranging from drop-in meetings with a cancer survivor serving as coordinator to educational and pedagogic class formats to intensive group psychotherapy (Spira, 1998). The style of facilitating groups depends on group format, patient make-up, stated goals, and the therapist's training (factors that are discussed in later chapters).

Differences Between the Current Protocol and Other Groups for Medically Ill Patients

Three fundamental styles of therapeutic intervention can be described, each of which may be suited to a different therapeutic population or group structure. The manner with which any topic is discussed can be deductive or didactically directed by the therapist, inductive facilitation with patient generated topics facilitated by therapists, or a balanced interaction between therapist and patients (see Table 3.2). Each has merit when used appropriately, and each is used in the model presented here.

TABLE 3.1

Characteristics of Groups Presenting for Various Purposes

Group population	Group characteristics	
	Presenting concern	Cognitive style
Community support groups	Heterogeneous	Heterogeneous
Relational–interpersonal	Heterogeneous	Homogenous
Psychological diagnosis	Homogenous	Homogenous
Common medical illness	Homogenous	Heterogeneous

Note. From "Understanding and Developing Psychotherapy Groups for Medically Ill Patients," by J. Spira, in *Group Psychotherapy for Medically Ill Patients* (p. 12), edited by J. Spira, 1997, New York: Guilford Press. Adapted with permission from Guilford Publishing © 1997.

DEDUCTIVE PROCESS

When the goal of a group is health education, the therapist serves primarily to give information. The therapist presents topics, so that patients obtain information helpful to them now or in the future. Specific readings or exercises may also be recommended. At its best, this approach uses sound educational principles, presenting information in the context of patients' lives, worldview, and motivational concerns so that each patient can best integrate the information into their lives in a way that works for them (Telch & Telch 1986). In the present model, we include the use of *The Breast Cancer Notebook: The Healing Power of Reflection* (Stan-

TABLE 3.2

Styles of Therapeutic Facilitation

Deductive	Interactive	Inductive
Lecture about set topics for education. May recommend exercises, readings, other resources.	Provide general information about set topics. Provide exercise to personalize for patients' specific situation. Facilitate discussion for integration of topic into patients' lives.	Discussion of any topic of concern raised by members is facilitated by the therapist to enable authentic communication, encourage life adjustment, provide group support, and promote active coping.

Note. From "Understanding and Developing Psychotherapy Groups for Medically Ill Patients," by J. Spira, in *Group Psychotherapy for Medically Ill Patients* (p. 6), edited by J. Spira, 1997, New York: Guilford Press. Copyright 1997 by Guilford Press. Reprinted by permission.

ton & Reed, 2002) and certain therapeutic exercises to stimulate exploration of patient concerns.

INDUCTIVE PROCESS

A more traditional form of group therapy occurs when therapists facilitate discussion of any topic that group members raise. Rather than presenting specific topics to be learned or practiced, the focus here is on facilitating the process of discussion, such that participants are speaking of issues in personal, specific, affective terms and are interacting with others to find active coping strategies to help them adjust to changing life circumstances (Spira, 1997a). In this approach, therapists rarely lecture or give advice. Nor do they generally give specific exercises to structure the interactions among patients. Instead, therapists facilitate discussion among participants by occasionally asking questions as needed to get patients back on track (Carkhuff, 2000; Egan, 1973; Yalom, 1985). When the discussion is going well, there is no need for therapists to speak at all. Because this approach can serve as a basis for all types of groups and styles of facilitation and is central to the model presented here, it is presented in some detail later on (see chapter 5, this volume).

INTERACTIVE PROCESS

In an approach that blends inductive and deductive processes, therapists facilitate patient interaction around certain topics, such as improving communication with medical personnel, adjusting to physical changes, and so on. Those using a cognitive–behavioral group format frequently follow this format (Spira, 1997c). A structured approach is most commonly used to balance psychoeducation, experience, and discussion, as shown in the following example:

- *Part 1*. Therapists present a particular topic, providing general information for 5 to 10 minutes.
- *Part 2*. Participants do a 10–20 minute exercise (e.g., paper and pencil, dyads, imagery) to personalize the exercise for their specific circumstances. This can be done in the group or, when time is limited, as homework.
- *Part 3*. Therapists facilitate a discussion about how these strategies can be implemented in one's life, touching on successes and barriers to successful implementation. They can ask leading questions about specific topics to structure a group discussion about a topic (e.g., "Let's go around the group and have each person tell us her biggest stressor when going for treatment"). The discussion usually lasts the rest of the meeting. (Examples of this approach are provided in Antoni, 1997; Fawzy et al., 1997; and Thoresen & Bracke, 1997.)

Self-help approaches to group treatment usually follow a psycho-educational approach that includes information sharing and skills acquisition. Although such approaches can be invaluable in explaining important information, they do little to address the emotional needs of patients. For this reason, in the current model we address patients' informational and emotional needs. A cognitive–behavioral approach to group psychotherapy minimizes lecturing or advice giving. Instead, it focuses on teaching skills and on reflecting on problems that occur in daily life.

The current approach contains psychoeducational, inductive, and interactive psychotherapeutic aspects. The psychoeducational aspect of this intervention emphasizes patient-centered self-guided access to educational material rather than didactic presentations by the therapist. This psychotherapeutic approach has an inductive, interpersonal emphasis supported with elements of cognitive therapy to assist in coping with treatment and adjusting to a new lifestyle. This combined approach is driven by two considerations: what cancer experts have identified as useful for patients to consider and what the patients themselves find important in their lives.

Clearly, differing goals of group therapy have different therapeutic emphases. The approach advocated here minimizes advice giving and maximizes experience through skill development and interpersonal exchange. Group therapy based on interpersonal difficulties emphasizes personality patterns that affect interpersonal relationships and the complementary early developmental relationships that serve to form one's personality. Therapy entails experiencing these conflicts in the group, with reflection about how these conflicts stem from one's personality style or early development. In contrast, our approach for women with breast cancer emphasizes directly experiencing ways of actively coping with existential and interpersonal conflicts through supportive interactions naturally arising in the group, without psychological interpretation or explanation (see Table 3.3). Early sessions are more structured, with therapists initially raising topics, whereas later sessions are more inductive as patients require less therapeutic input.

Influences on the Therapeutic Style Recommended in This Model

The specific therapeutic and philosophical approaches that influence the current approach are briefly discussed below.

Comparing Educational, Cognitive–Behavioral, and Social–Emotional Supportive Group Therapy

Type of group	Therapeutic emphasis		
	Advice	Focus	Experience
Educational	Mostly given	Information	Incidental
Cognitive– behavioral	Sometimes given	Skill-oriented	Reflection about problem occurring throughout one's life; practice specific skills in special exercises
Group therapy for persons with psycho- social issues	Rarely given	Personality patterns affecting inter- personal rela- tionships (and vice versa)	Directly experience interpersoal style of relating, w/therapeu- tic reflection about these in- teractions to reveal patterns
Group therapy for persons with cancer	Rarely given	Existential suppor- tive coping	Directly experience alternative ways of active coping through interactions naturallty arising in group, w/o interpretation

Note. From "Group Psychotherapy for Persons With Cancer," by J. Spira, in *Psychooncology* (p. 708), edited by J. Holland, 1998, New York: Oxford University Press. Copyright © 1998 by Oxford University Press. Re- printed by permission.

BASIC COUNSELING FORMAT

Psychotherapy typically involves the use of active listening to support patients' expression of their experience (Carkhuff, 2000; Corey, 2000; Egan, 1973). The approach advocated here is no exception. Rapport is established through active listening on the part of the therapist and other group members to show support for the patients' expression of their experience. However, whereas our model recommends establish- ing a foundation of rapport, it also gently challenges patients to explore alternative ways of viewing their situation, expressing their feelings, coping with problems, and considering what is most meaningful in their lives. Thus, beyond laying a foundation of simple rapport, therapists encourage expression in personal, specific, and affective terms (see Ex- hibit 3.1).

INTERPERSONAL THERAPY

An essential aspect of our approach draws from the traditional inter- personal therapy approach to group facilitation. Breaking with Sigmund Freud, Alfred Adler focused on the development of self in relationship

The Role of Therapists

The role of therapists is to

- establish rapport,
- engage in reflective listening (especially when others do not),
- ask questions rather than give answers, and
- ask questions which help group members to express themselves in personal, specific, and affective terms.

to one's interaction with others (Adler & Brett, 1998). This was later elaborated by object relations theorists. Psychotherapeutic intervention focused on reestablishing an intimate relationship in one's adulthood in hopes that this would help to reshape one's self in a way more congruent with current circumstances. Carl Rogers (1961) attempted to facilitate a more positive acceptance of one's self through establishing an accepting relationship in therapy. Harry Stack Sullivan (1953) emphasized the therapeutic relationship as well as the interpersonal relationships in patients' past and current life. Gerald Klerman et al. (1984) developed an abbreviated version of interpersonal therapy focusing on current interpersonal relationships in a person's life, but largely ignoring the interpersonal relationship occurring within the therapy session and in the patient's formative years. Irvin Yalom (1985) has applied many of these principles to the group therapy format, emphasizing interpersonal relations within the group. The approach advocated here uses the power of group support and acceptance to help cancer patients explore and accept their changing interpersonal relations on self-image and social functioning (see Exhibit 3.2).

EXISTENTIAL PSYCHOTHERAPY

Traditionally, existential psychotherapy has been less "technique oriented" than a set of guiding principles for conducting therapy (Spira, 1997a, 2000; Yalom, 1980). Existential philosophers emphasize the role of significant personal crisis as central to recognizing and going beyond one's habitual conditioned existence to live more fully. This occurs when one can express and act in a way congruent with what yields greatest personal meaning, purpose, and value in one's life. (See, e.g., works by Soren Kierkegaard, 1944, Friedrich Nietzsche, 1967, and Martin Heidegger, 1962.)

Individual therapists have emphasized various aspects of existential philosophy in attempting to assist patients to live more fully in the face of crisis. Karl Jaspers (1913/1994) and Binswanger (1946/1958) em-

---

EXHIBIT 3.2

Fostering Interpersonal Development

When necessary to foster interpersonal development, group members are asked to

- relate to the therapist,
- relate to each other,
- discuss past relationships that might bear on their current concerns,
- discuss current relationships, and
- discuss future optimal relationships.

---

phasized allowing patients to express their concerns within their life context rather than categorizing them into deductive categories for the convenience of the therapists. Irvin Yalom (1980) and James Bugental (1978) have suggested that "staying in the moment" in therapy helps patients notice the way they "cover up" their fear of dying by "fleeing" into conventional habits. Therapy helps them to tolerate the inevitability of death, thereby better accepting (rather than fleeing from) everyday life. Experientially oriented therapists (e.g., Gendlin, 1979; Maslow, 1968; Perls, 1969) have emphasized growth in terms of peak or integrated moments in which one can function as fully as possible. Martin E. P. Seligman (1998) referred to this emphasis on optimal functioning rather than correcting pathology as "positive psychology."

The approach taken here uses all these aspects as guiding principles throughout the therapeutic process to assist group members to adjust to and go beyond their current situation by letting go of past fixed self-images and focusing on how they can develop greatest meaning, purpose, and value in their current and future lives. Although no one wants cancer, this crisis presents an opportunity for reflection and growth (see Exhibit 3.3).

COGNITIVE THERAPY

The cognitive approach, developed by Albert Ellis (1962), William Glasser (1965), and others, helps patients recognize and alter cognitive distortions that affect how one thinks, feels, and acts. The model states that one's worldview (one's beliefs and assumptions about the way the world operates) leads to a specific pattern of thoughts, emotions, physiological responses, and behaviors. Although one's worldview (e.g., "I must do everything myself") may be initially accurate (as a child, one's parents were not around to support activities), it tends to be overused ("I can't rely on anyone to help me"), with negative consequences to health and well-being (finding it difficult to go to a doctor when feeling a breast

---

EXHIBIT 3.3

Fostering Existential Development

Therapists allow group members to

- describe their situation and express their concerns in their own terms and with their own values, allowing for rich diversity within the group;
- develop the ability to focus primarily on each moment, with occasional reflection of relevant past experience and contemplation of desired future; and
- adjust to the situation at hand, by exploring ways to enhance meaning, purpose, and value in their lives.

---

lump, being unable to ask for assistance in going to radiotherapy even though it makes one too ill to drive, etc.; see Exhibit 3.4). The cognitive therapist challenges patients' assumptions about life. This can be accomplished in a variety of ways, for instance by asking the patient how this belief was formed or by drawing on other patients in the group for alternative ways of viewing a situation or reacting to it.

Challenging beliefs that limit patients' quality of life and possibly their compliance with medical recommendations can help them recognize their limitations and begin to consider alternatives. Such an approach has been found to be helpful for people whose personality factors are clearly related to disease progression, such as cardiac patients with Type A behavior. However, for patients with breast cancer, especially in the first 6 months following diagnosis, it is more important to address issues of coping with treatment and adjusting to a new lifestyle than confronting lifelong patterns of behavior and underlying beliefs that are not significantly influencing their current cancer-related situation. Individual personality characteristics that affect coping and adjustment can

---

EXHIBIT 3.4

Identifying Restrictive Beliefs

Typically, beliefs that may result in suboptimal coping with breast cancer can be found in statements such as

- I have to do everything myself.
- I need to be in complete control.
- I can't let myself be scared (or sad or worried).
- I have no control.
- I can't let myself enjoy what I've got.
- I can't let my family know how worried I am.

---

be gently confronted by establishing a milieu in which group members can listen to the way others manage their lives, so that direct therapeutic challenge is not often required. For the most part, the cognitive therapy approach is a secondary consideration in this model of group treatment. Yet it can be especially useful when patients feel "stuck" in coping with some aspect of their lives as cancer patients.

COGNITIVE–BEHAVIOR THERAPY

CBT is a simplified version of cognitive therapy that tends to use specific techniques for specifically identified problems. The approach has been used effectively for major depression, phobias, anxiety and panic disorders, and specific aspects of personality disorders (Beck et al., 1979). Specific skills are emphasized to counter habitual cognitive, affective, and behavioral reactions in situations that may trigger maladaptive behaviors. CBT has flourished under managed care environments because it offers specific techniques for specific symptom management and specific psychological factors directly related to them. However, although CBT is useful for reducing identifiable maladaptive behaviors, it lacks an inductive approach to uncovering patient concerns, especially fundamental, generalized existential considerations. Furthermore, the current approach views most patients' responses as normal and natural reactions to a life-threatening events, best dealt with through providing an understanding environment that allows for open expression of fears and hopes. The present model uses some cognitive–behavioral tools for reducing distress, but for the most part it attempts to inductively elicit deeper patient concerns and feelings (see Exhibit 3.5).

Principles of Group Therapy for Medically Ill Patients

Presented below is a brief summary of the therapeutic process and the content of topics discussed in this protocol. In subsequent chapters we present the way groups are structured and an in-depth presentation of facilitating the group process.

The psychotherapeutic process used in the groups emphasizes four major aspects of therapist involvement. In all cases, the therapist asks questions (rather than provides information) and only intervenes as necessary to keep the group on track. In general, therapists invite group members to express their concerns but never challenge them aggressively. Therapists also limit their interaction with any individual to just a few questions, so that group members can engage one another.

EXHIBIT 3.5

Fostering Active Coping

Therapists help group members to actively cope with their situation by asking questions which prompt members to

- recognize fixed patterns of thinking (beliefs, distortions) that limit their ability to cope with a current problem,
- consider alternative ways of approaching their problem, and
- actively practice new solutions between group meetings, reporting back to the group their experiences with this new approach.

1. Interpersonal support is provided through the therapists' establishing both individual and group rapport. This is accomplished by using active listening skills and exhibiting unconditional respect for group members and their experience. Therapists also ensure that there is fundamental mutual respect among group members, with all members able to express their personal experiences, thoughts, and feelings without criticism. Therapists encourage interaction among group participants rather than merely inviting a series of individual expressions. Group members are also encouraged to interact outside of the group sessions if they so choose.

2. Authentic expression is elicited through the therapist asking questions of an individual or the group that help to make sure that statements group members make are personal (rather than solely about other people), specific (rather than focusing on generalizations and abstract ideas), and affective (rather than purely intellectual). By asking questions of group members that lead them to make personal, specific, and affectively rich statements, group members are able to explore their condition in ways that feel honest and integrated to them. Negative thoughts and feelings are not avoided; they are as fully discussed as group members are able to tolerate.

3. Active coping strategies are developed through discussing what can be controlled and accepting what cannot be controlled. When encountering passive helplessness on the part of group members, therapists attempt to elicit active behaviors and attitudes from them by discussing alternative ways of coping with the situation. Furthermore, patients are encouraged to think about what one can do rather than what one cannot act on.

4. Adjusting to present circumstances is facilitated through gently and positively challenging basic assumptions that tend to restrict group members from fully engaging in their lives in light of their

new circumstances. Existential aspects of members' concerns are emphasized, eliciting from them ways that the illness has prompted ways of living fully in the face of dying; reprioritizing activities; and finding maximum meaning, value, and purpose in their lives. Ways in which members' self-image limits their potential for development are explored. Therapists encourage discussion of various ways that individuals might enrich their lives, resisting attempts to impose a belief that there is only one way to find fulfillment in life.

Topics are elicited inductively from the group. That is, therapists do not typically present topics to be discussed but rather allow group members to discuss whatever concerns they currently have. There may be a desire to discuss issues of relevance that arise from the material in *The Breast Cancer Notebook* or to continue a discussion from the previous week. The role of the therapist is to ensure that whatever is being discussed is expressed authentically, within an atmosphere of interpersonal support, with an eye toward improving group members' active coping and adjustment to present circumstances.

The Therapeutic Role

Although group psychotherapy for women with breast cancer appears to be a subspecialty of group psychotherapy, facilitation with this group of patients in fact requires more breadth of training than working with many other groups. Therapists should be familiar with psychotherapeutic methods including cognitive therapy (active coping skills), behavioral skills (relaxation, pain management), facilitation of social support and emotional expression (as outlined above), and existential considerations (Yalom, 1980). Whereas training and experience in these psychotherapeutic methods are essential, additional training in group therapy is also a prerequisite for effective group treatment (Yalom, 1985). Finally, experience with medically ill patients is also useful. Until sufficient experience is obtained, leading groups with an experienced therapist can serve as excellent on-the-job training. At the very least, these criteria should be met between two cotherapists.

The therapists' most important function is to create a safe environment that fosters both the expression of patient concerns and the process of positive change that can result from this. In the context of this therapeutic approach, the role of the therapist is to accept, reflect, and encourage expression of often-difficult thoughts and feelings. Through this process, the therapist helps the group members tolerate and explore their fears and frustrations. These feelings may seem particularly overwhelming to members when they relate to the threat of mortality and the shadow this threat casts over every area of their lives. The therapist must facilitate group members' provision of mutual support for such expression, by helping group members to tolerate and reflect feelings of others even though therapists own feelings may be triggered by sad disclosures.

THERAPISTS AS "EXPERTS"

Therapists should not be "content experts" giving advice on treatment or life issues. Whether facilitators are oncologists or nurses serving as medical experts or psychologists or social workers giving advice about lifestyle improvement, their expertise tends to shift the dynamic of the group from an active development of its own culture and process of exploration to the more passive stance of information seeking. If the therapist has relevant information that appears to be needed, or if external experts are brought into the group, such presentations should be as brief as possible or even deferred until the group meeting is over.

PERSONAL DISCLOSURE AND INVOLVEMENT

Therapist disclosure of personal distress is typically not a good idea, because members like an anchor of stability in the group. On the other hand, therapists who disclose that they are also concerned with many of these same issues can show group members that these are issues of intimate concern rather than an academic exercise for the therapist. Occasionally, therapists have had cancer or a serious illness themselves. Even without the experience of serious illness, most therapists have experienced the death or serious illness of a loved one or have considered that they could be hit by a car at any moment, and such reflection can help their emotional maturity. Yet the group is formed for the group members, not therapists, and as such therapists should not use the group to receive personal help or attempt to dictate a single method to follow. Disclosure of such material should be made carefully and sensitively and only when there is a clear therapeutic purpose to the disclosure and the therapist has a specific treatment goal in mind related to the group material at the time the disclosure is made. Often, group members (particularly women) ask therapists if they have had cancer quite early in the group. So it is a good idea to be prepared to handle this issue.

Therapists should be careful not to express their distress in the group (although a natural rapport of sadness or happiness shows authenticity on the part of the therapist). Nevertheless, paying attention to one's emotional reactions can mirror what others in the group may be feeling. Sadness, discomfort, or irritability may be shared by many members, and these feelings can be discussed. To determine the fine line between unusual personal reactions to a member or the group and feelings that are common to the group, debriefing with a cotherapist can be especially helpful.

Working with cancer patients can be extremely rewarding, as long as therapists are willing to confront issues of death and dying or strong negative emotions in an open and honest way. Fear of dealing with such issues and feelings may lead the therapist to rush away from group members' distress, which in turn may lead the members to flee from their own emotions. It is normal for therapists to want to rush away from strong negative emotions and thoughts or to rescue the distressed patient and therefore take care of their own distress. However, if they can tolerate the discussion and expressions, then the members would be better able to tolerate their experiences and cope more effectively with them. A balance between accepting negative thoughts and feelings and considering ways to moderate them is far more effective than rushing into positive solutions, which can be a form of denial of the feelings and avoidance of issues the member lives with constantly.

Group facilitation by a pair of therapists is discussed in chapter 4.

THERAPIST TRAINING FOR RESEARCH PURPOSES

Training in our protocol for research purposes must take a rigorous approach. Earlier breast cancer training manuals for research purposes have been used in three phases. The first phase entails study of the training manual. The second phase includes a 15-hour workshop to discuss and practice the principles outlined in the manual. An important component of this workshop has been the review and discussion of videotaped vignettes from actual breast cancer groups. Whenever possible, we recommend obtaining such video training. The third phase entails ongoing supervision. We have found the review of audiotapes or videotapes of selected group therapy sessions to be highly effective. Feedback regarding clinical strategies and adherence to the treatment approach that is provided to the cotherapists in a timely manner is essential for establishing and maintaining a high quality of therapeutic skill. Supervising therapists may request more or fewer tapes as needed to facilitate further monitoring and feedback.

Group Structure and Content | 4

efore launching into specific therapeutic interventions, the overall group structure will be discussed.

Planning and Forming a Group

STRUCTURE

We recommend that groups meet weekly for 16 consecutive weeks (with the exception of holidays), with each session lasting 2 hours. Traditional therapy groups more typically meet for 90 minutes, but 2 hours are required to incorporate the structural elements described below while leaving sufficient time for open discussion and exploration of issues.

Each group member should be asked to commit to the entire 16 sessions, with all group members beginning at the first group. This is called a *closed group* and allows for the greatest degree of development for individuals in the group and the group as a whole. Although "drop-in" groups are appropriate for some settings and treatment methods, we believe that intermittent attendance is disruptive for the group bonding that is an important part of the approach described here.

The only real disadvantage of a closed-group program arises when there is an urgent need to get a patient into a group, without waiting until a new group is formed. For example, we would not advise requesting that a woman newly diagnosed with breast cancer who is experiencing acute distress wait several weeks for a new group to begin. Many comprehensive programs offer shorter term drop-in groups to accommodate patients in these situations and others who prefer this format. Such brief drop-in groups can accommodate people with any type of cancer diagnosis, and they generally focus on providing some initial support. Drop-in groups often focus on helping patients to obtain specific information about cancer and treatment and to connect to community resources, and they may also provide patients an opportunity to learn basic relaxation skills. These groups are not intended to provide the depth of experience of longer term closed groups such as the one described in this manual. Instead, they serve a valuable function in crisis management and serve as a "holding" group until the 16-week group becomes available.

GROUP COMPOSITION

We highly recommend that groups be as homogenous as possible. Patients experiencing a first occurrence should meet separately from those experiencing a recurrence or those with metastatic disease. Although mixed-stage groups can be conducted with benefit to the group members, they are much more difficult to manage and require considerable skill and training on the part of the therapists to ensure that the broad range of issues involved is openly discussed. A woman who recently had a lumpectomy may be reluctant to discuss issues related to dating when there is another member facing a painful procedure to save her life or slow the encroachment of metastasis. Yet both are important issues for these group members. In addition, women with a first occurrence of disease typically try to cope with the treatment, put their illness behind them, and get on with their lives, whereas women with recurrent disease may have little chance of putting their disease behind them. However, it is generally better to offer a mixed-stage group than no group at all, as long as therapists are able to focus on common themes and allow each member to express her concerns without fear of these being considered too "petty" or too "upsetting" to bring up in the group. (See chapter 8 for more discussion on groups for people with various diagnoses and stages of illness.)

GROUP RECRUITMENT

Groups for breast cancer patients are frequently offered in treatment settings in hospitals and clinics. They can also be offered through the private offices of a breast surgeon or an oncologist. It is important to discuss the group program with the physicians involved in the treatment of patients likely to be good candidates for the group. However, the best sources of referrals are likely to be clinic nurses, receptionists, and other office staff, so it is useful to meet with these individuals separately to explain the program and discuss what types of patients might be appropriate candidates. Flyers, announcements, or brochures can be placed in waiting and treatment areas, but our experience is that these are not sufficient without support from clinic staff. In general, the better the therapist is integrated into the treatment setting, the more likely that patients will be referred and that a group program will be successful over time. Therapists should consider ways in which they can be helpful to clinic or office staff. For example, a therapist who is knowledgeable about relaxation techniques might provide an in-service training on this topic for nurses in the chemotherapy room. (Recruitment issues are discussed at greater length in chapter 8.)

GROUP SIZE

Our experience is that optimal group size is between 8 and 10 members. Groups with more than 12 members are difficult to manage, even with two therapists, and less assertive members may have difficulty negotiating the attention they need. Very small groups (6 or fewer) may begin to lose the richness of group interaction and may be particularly difficult to hold if 1 or 2 members miss a particular session. However, we recognize that in some settings it may be difficult to recruit sufficient numbers of patients for a larger group. We successfully have run groups with as few as 3 members. With groups of such small size, it is critical that consistent attendance be negotiated with all group members.

PREGROUP INTAKE INTERVIEW

We recommend that one or both of the cotherapists meet initially with each group candidate for a general intake interview. These interviews can serve several important functions. First, a preliminary meeting helps to form a bond between the therapist and group member. Such a bond can assist the group member in entering the group, reducing her anxiety, and helping her to believe that the group will be beneficial. It may also help the candidate to tolerate a delay in getting the group started. Second, an initial interview helps the therapists to learn about what the candidate wishes to get out of the group. Third, it allows for an initial discussion of the nature, format, and focus of the group and whether the candidate's needs and expectations are likely to be met. Fourth, it allows therapists to identify individuals with sufficiently high levels of distress or disturbance that they should be referred for immediate individual treatment. In these cases, the group is frequently an appropriate form of treatment after initial stabilization or as an adjunct to individual treatment. Finally, the initial interview allows the therapists an opportunity to identify and refer those relatively few individuals with serious mental health conditions for whom the group may not be the most appropriate form of treatment.

It is important to ask the patient what makes her interested in joining the group and what she hopes to gain from participating. Other topics that the therapists should consider asking about during the initial interview include the time and circumstances of diagnosis, past and planned treatment, current emotional and psychological functioning, preexisting and current life stressors, family and living circumstances, and prior experience with psychotherapy and groups. It can be useful to ask about the patient's responses to prior difficult experiences to get a sense of coping resources and style. It is also important to ask about the availability of support in the patient's life and to get a sense of who provides it. When asking about the presence of a primary partner, the therapists should be sensitive to the possibility of lesbian partnerships that may go unmentioned. The level of experienced support in the primary relationship as well as any difficulties in the relationship should be briefly assessed. Relationship issues may be more easily disclosed in the one-on-one setting of the pregroup interview. The patient is then more likely to bring this material into the group because she has already discussed it with the therapists.

If the therapists determine on the basis of the initial interview that the woman is a good candidate and is appropriate for the group, we recommend that she be given a copy of *The Breast Cancer Notebook: The Healing Power of Reflection* (Stanton & Reed, 2002) at that time. *The Breast Cancer Notebook* has been developed as an integral part of this treatment program, although it is certainly possible to run successful groups without using it if the therapists prefer. If the notebook is used, therapists should take the time to be familiar with its contents before giving it to group members. The notebook attempts to provide a structure and self-guided process through which each woman participating in the group can assess and reflect on the impact that breast cancer has had on specific areas of her life. This exploration is intended both to expand on and to enrich the discussion during group sessions. The notebook contains chapters that focus on important topics for breast cancer patients (e.g., coping with side effects, family and friends, work, body image and sexuality) and provides educational material, additional resources, and questions intended as a guide for personal reflection regarding each topic. The early chapters of the notebook are specifically keyed to the early sessions of the group, as is described below. Additional information about integrating *The Breast Cancer Notebook* into the group therapy is provided later in this chapter and in chapter 7.

When giving *The Breast Cancer Notebook* to the prospective group member, the therapists should briefly review its content and purpose. The therapists should tell the group member that this information is not being given as "homework" but because it may provide a very useful resource. The group member should be asked to read through chapter 1, "Finding Your Way," and to think about the questions at the end of the chapter before the group begins. In addition to having both informational and therapeutic value in its own right, the notebook can provide a useful bridge to the group and what will be considered in the group until the group actually begins.

GUIDELINES FOR GROUP MEMBERS

The frame of the group—that is, the boundaries and mutual agreements regarding participation—is a critical part of the group's effectiveness. The boundaries of the group members' mutual contract encourage them to treat the group with seriousness and create a basis for mutual trust. Although this frame is similar to that used in many other group approaches, some aspects merit specific consideration here. In addition, several structural elements are used to encourage a sense of safety and interconnection among group members and to facilitate the therapeutic goals of the group.

The first group meeting should include a description of the following aspects of the treatment.

Time

Group sessions are held weekly for 2 hours. Although many groups are conducted for 90 minutes, 2 hours are required to incorporate the structural elements described below while leaving sufficient time for open discussion and exploration. The importance for the group of being on time is discussed, and therapists should indicate that the group will begin and end at the stated hour.

Attendance

Therapists should discuss the importance of making an effort to attend every session, given the time-limited nature of the group, although tolerance and understanding for each woman's individual circumstances that may force her to miss a particular session should be conveyed. Members are asked to notify the group in advance if they plan to miss a session. If something arises at the last moment, members are asked to call one of the therapists before the session. If a member calls one of the therapists to notify the group of her absence, the therapist will ask the member to indicate what she would like the therapist to tell the other group members regarding her absence. This information is conveyed at the beginning of group sessions. This helps to minimize what may otherwise be very unnecessary worry regarding the absent members' health. Furthermore, this structure communicates the view that each member is accountable to the group, not the therapists. Overall, being accountable for every session reinforces the commitment to attend sessions, even when one might not feel up to it. Our experience tells us that, even when they are fatigued or feeling "down," group members almost always feel better for having attended.

Confidentiality

The confidentiality of personal material revealed in group sessions is handled in much the same way as in other therapy groups. Additional aspects of this issue, however, are important in groups for women with breast cancer. Individuals in patients' social networks and places of employment may be unaware of the breast cancer diagnosis, and there may be negative consequences to inadvertent disclosure by others. Furthermore, it is possible that group members have overlapping social networks. Therapists should remind group members to be careful when talking to anyone outside the group and not to discuss any other member in a manner that would allow her to be identified. The possibility that they may encounter one another in public places or socially should also be discussed, and guidelines for handling such occasions should be provided.

For example, if meeting outside the group, a member should not bring up an issue about another member, unless that member expresses a desire to discuss it herself. In other words, whatever one brings up in the group stays in the group, unless the member indicates she personally wishes to discuss it with others. In this way, members can feel safe expressing whatever feelings and thoughts they wish, without fear of unintended consequences that might ensue.

Socializing

Members should also be told that, unlike some other forms of group therapy, they are free to associate outside the group. They may choose to exchange phone numbers and to see one another between sessions. It is important, however, that these meetings not be kept secret from the others. If members see one another outside the group, they must report this to the group and let the group know what they did when they got together. It is best for the therapists to adopt an encouraging though relatively neutral attitude toward social interactions among members outside the group. If members choose to exchange telephone numbers or to organize get-togethers, they should initiate and manage these tasks themselves. Therapists should also make sure that the group is respectful of members who do not wish to participate in telephone lists or social contacts between groups. Every patient's situation is unique, and contact that may feel helpful and supportive to some members may make other members feel pressured or intruded on. If necessary, the therapists should normalize such reactions to make sure that members who have a greater need for privacy or separateness do not feel ostracized and to help other members not to perceive this as personal rejection.

Use of Cotherapists

The use of cotherapists is an important aspect of this model of treatment. Although a smaller group of 6–8 participants can be managed by a single therapist, we recommend that two therapists facilitate patient groups whenever feasible. This is particularly important when group size exceeds 8 members, because the cotherapist helps to ensure appropriate attention to every group member's issues.

Cotherapists may come from a variety of backgrounds, including psychology, psychiatry, nursing, social work, and even oncology. We suggest that cotherapists complement each other in terms of background, orientation, and experience whenever possible. Between them, the cotherapists should have the following characteristics:

- group experience
- psychotherapy training
- experience working with cancer patients (or at least with other medical populations).

If possible, at least one therapist should be a woman.

Although neither of us is a woman, we have not found this to be a handicap in the many groups for breast cancer patients we have led. This is in part because we have solicited the help of female therapists whenever possible and we used specific therapeutic devices. For example, when challenged with "How can you possibly understand what it is like to be a _____ (e.g., diabetic, alcoholic, migraine sufferer, breast cancer patient)?" we reply with "Can you help me to understand your experiences of living with this problem?"

We appreciate that institutions may often impose economic limitations on the ability of two licensed health care professionals to provide group therapy together. Yet the presence of two therapists for 2 hours per week can in fact save time and money for an organization. For example, patients are less likely to make unnecessary medical visits if the group is helping them to manage anxiety and is providing information and support. Participation in the group may also help patients to keep necessary medical appointments they may have been avoiding, thereby improving the outcomes of medical treatment. Thus, the presence of two therapists offers the institution a great deal of value for a small investment. In teaching settings, it can often be arranged that the therapist pair can include a mentor and a trainee. In such cases, the cotherapists may have to work to overcome their own feelings about the power differential between them so that this does not affect their capacity to function as equal partners in the group.

Therapists who work well together enrich the group and are of great value to the group process. There is so much to keep in mind during the course of a group—changing topics, getting back to a member on an important point not pursued earlier, tracking themes, tracking processes, attending to silent members, following up on an emotion that may have begun to emerge with a member at an earlier time—that two perspectives are helpful. The use of cotherapists can help to allow for greater complexity of material to emerge in the group as the two therapists track and respond to different aspects of the group's content and dynamics. Two therapists can complement one another in a variety of ways and may fill different functions at different times based on their individual skills, sensitivities, and experience.

Typically, cotherapists find that it is helpful to share difficult tasks. For example, cotherapists might track different processes in the group. One therapist might follow the thread of the conversation among the active members, helping to keep the group on one important topic for a while longer (especially if one member begins to introduce a new topic before others are ready to leave the first topic). The other therapist, meanwhile, might recognize and draw into the conversation more silent members, asking them if they can relate to the issues brought up by others. One therapist might be better at tracking the topic, whereas the other therapist might be better at recognizing and helping to draw out affect. As a cotherapy relationship develops, this type of give and take tends to become more fluid and spontaneous. Initially, it may require more discussion and planning.

Therapists should be cautious that they do not talk one after the other and end up dominating a discussion. They should allow space for one another to take the lead with a member or a theme, with the other serving to pitch in only briefly with a clarification only if needed. In general, the therapists together should speak far less than the members of the group. Sometimes the therapists may disagree regarding a particular viewpoint or recommendation. Such disagreements can actually be useful for the group and should be handled directly, openly, and respectfully. The cotherapy relationship can provide group members with a model of a fully communicative relationship that may contain both support and disagreement.

Cotherapists also provide two distinct therapeutic figures with whom group members may form differing relationships. Some group members are likely to be noticeably more connected with one therapist than with the other. The presence of at least one female therapist appears to be particularly helpful in making group members feel that their experiences as women can be understood and often seems to facilitate expressions of emotion related to grief and loss. Male–female cotherapist pairs may offer a particularly rich context for the group, because male and female therapists may attract different sets of reactions from members and stimulate discussion of different sets of issues. This may be based in part on transferential responses related to the therapists, and such responses are not a primary focus of treatment, and making explicit the dynamics that may underlie the symbolic use of the cotherapists is generally not relevant to the goals of the group. Thus, therapists need to tolerate being used as symbolic figures by group members who are working through issues relevant to their own lives.

Following each session, it is important for the cotherapists to allow plenty of time for debriefing and planning of the next session. Specific suggestions for debriefing are included at the end of this chapter.

Group Format

Throughout the 16 weeks of the therapy group, each group session includes the following basic elements: Opening Relaxation, Check-In, Group Discussion, Check-Out, and Closing Relaxation. The basic elements and timeline for a "typical" group session are shown in Table 4.1. These basic elements become part of a group routine, contributing to

TABLE 4.1

Format for Regular Group Meetings

Minutes into group	Process	Duration (approximate)
0	Close door	5 minutes
	Begin Opening Relaxation	
5	Check-In	15 minutes
20	Group Discussion	65 minutes
80	Signal end of meeting approaching	
90	Check-Out	15 minutes
105	Review next section of *Breast Cancer Notebook*	10 minutes
	Inquire about planned absences	
110	Closing Relaxation	10 minutes

the development of a group culture and a sense of the group as a safe container for group members' feelings and issues. Each of these elements is described in more detail in the following sections.

OPENING RELAXATION

The opening of each group session is marked by a 3- to 5-minute period of relaxation. The purpose of Opening Relaxation is to help participants shift focus from the activity of daily life to their own inner experience and to mark a transition into the group space. At the beginning of a group, the Opening Relaxation exercise serves to

- signal the formal start of the session;
- help calm members' minds after a busy commute to the group;
- bring the group together with a common, shared, and intimate experience; and
- teach a relaxation skill useful for reducing anxiety, assisting sleep, and improving one's ability to cope with oncotherapies.

The Opening Relaxation exercise is approximately 5 minutes long and should be geared toward self-comforting and mental calming. Opening Relaxation often begins with simple sensate focusing. Building on physical sensations that participants may notice (e.g., feelings of warmth that may be allowed to spread, muscle tension that can be released), therapists invite participants to allow themselves to become more relaxed and more comfortable. Participants may be invited to become aware of any thoughts and feelings or to allow new ones to surface. These may simply be noted in the context of physical relaxation and comfort. Group members may be invited to consider whether discussion of any of these thoughts and feelings might help them or the group.

As groups become more practiced with relaxation techniques, the Opening Relaxation exercise can also permit participants to experiment with the opening of feelings and thoughts that might otherwise be too insistent to tolerate. In the context of opening relaxation, these feelings and thoughts can be accessed in a more controlled manner, thereby reducing tension. During later weeks of the group, the Opening Relaxation exercise can be used as an opportunity to note the concerns that are on a participant's mind, allowing these to surface and even using them as a way to begin the discussion that day. In selecting relaxation techniques, the therapists should be aware that sometimes exercises that focus on the chest (e.g., the rise and fall of the chest during breathing) may be uncomfortable for breast cancer patients because this area may be uncomfortable, scarred, or a locus of emotional sensitivity.

Several weeks into the group, it is useful for the cotherapists to begin a brief discussion of group members' experience of the various relaxation techniques that have been used—which ones work well, which ones do not, the extent to which group members are finding them helpful outside the group, and so on—if such a discussion has not arisen spontaneously during the group. This feedback can be used to modify the relaxation techniques that are selected. After the ritual and the relaxation techniques used are well-established, it is often helpful and fun to allow interested members to lead some of the relaxation exercises. This helps to enhance members' sense of control, mastery, and self-efficacy in relation to the relaxation techniques, encouraging them to practice the techniques at home between group meetings.

Exhibit 4.1 describes a simple breath-oriented meditation that can be both calming of the mind and comforting to the body. It is the type of simple and brief exercise often used for Opening Relaxation.

Examples of other simple yet powerful relaxation and meditation exercises are contained in chapter 5 and in the Appendix.

CHECK-IN

The Opening Relaxation exercise is followed by a brief Check-In by each member of the group. The purposes of Check-In include providing each member with the opportunity to let other group members know about any crisis or pressing need for which she needs group time and attention. Furthermore, Check-In helps each member to focus and begin to use the group session by identifying, articulating, structuring, and prioritizing feelings or issues with which she is dealing or wishes to discuss with others.

Check-In also helps all group members to be aware of and to listen to one another. Going around the room, each member takes 1–2 minutes to describe to the group members any issues or feelings that have been important for her during the past week. Members are encouraged to talk about any feelings they have about being in the group session on that particular day and any thoughts and feelings that have been triggered by the session the week before. Members may also bring up any thoughts, feelings, questions, or needs for discussion that were stimulated by their reading assignment in *The Breast Cancer Notebook*.

Check-In is also an appropriate time to comment or inquire about any group members who are missing. (It is generally most helpful to do this before going around the room, because members may be preoccupied or unsettled by unexplained absences.) Whereas some members may have announced a planned absence (e.g., travel, appointment) in advance, others may be absent unexpectedly. Showing honest concern for them helps the group know that they are cared for and this in turn supports better attendance and notification of planned absences. Therapists should let group members know that they plan to call anyone who is unexpectedly absent and check on her welfare.

EXHIBIT 4.1

Sample Opening Relaxation Exercise

1. Sit comfortably in your chair, with your back erect, eyes open and looking downward, and your hands resting on your belly. (Note: Eyes may be open or closed, depending on each member's preference. It is useful to practice both ways.) Whenever you notice your attention being pulled by thoughts (creating your own visual images, conversations, feelings), just note that distraction, let it go, and gently return your attention to what is right here. Do not control your breath but instead simply observe its effortless activity.
2. Notice the air flowing into and out of your nose and throat. Notice how the temperature changes from the inhale to the exhale, the different places the air touches, and the different qualities of the air against the nose and throat. Count 10 more breaths flowing into and out from your nose.
3. Notice how your rib cage moves forward and back, expands out to the sides, and even expands into your back with each breath. Find the point in the middle of your body from which this expansion occurs and to which it releases. Count 10 more times as the breath expands from this location and returns to it.
4. Notice your belly gently rocking your hands to and fro. Feel the gentle warmth of your body, and the effortlessness with which it rocks your hands. Count 10 more times that your body rocks your hands forward and back.
5. Finally, experience in silence the breath effortlessly expanding and releasing your body. As you breathe in, feel as if you are accepting everything you see, hear, and feel into the center of your breath. With every exhalation, feel as if you are giving yourself completely away to what you see, hear, and feel.
6. When you are ready, begin noticing your chest rising with each inhale. Let your breath come a little fuller into that inhale, raising your chest a little bit higher. Now, with the next inhale, let your eyes and eyelids rise up with that breath, all the way up to the ceiling. Then, refocus on the room; feeling calm, clear, focused, and ready to begin the group.

Therapists should make explicit to members that the purpose of Check-In is not simply to recite the events of the week or to give a general appraisal of one's mood over the week; rather, it is a time to identify issues and themes that are important to them. Members are told that its purpose is to take stock of what is going on with everyone so that the group can offer support and discuss relevant issues during the session. Members should feel free to mention that they want to continue discussing a particular issue after the go-around, and therapists may want to inquire further about certain issues after the go-around as well. Group members may have equally important concerns. If one group member is worried about a recurrence, and another group member is concerned with an upcoming family event, both issues may be equally important to the group member herself. Thus, therapists should track each group member's concerns and offer an opportunity for her to talk about her issues during the session. Common themes often are raised, and they form the basis of that session's discussion.

During Check-In, other group members and the therapists sometimes ask questions to clarify or deepen the issues and feelings presented, but the therapists also communicate that major exploration of specific issues will wait until all group members have checked in. For example, a therapist may tell a member who begins to engage in an extended expression or exploration of a particular issue that this might be something important to discuss with the whole group later during the session. Therapists should not, in general, abandon the structure of Check-In to attend to a particular member's material. Because each member is heard from, the process of Check-In helps less assertive members who have pressing issues to identify their need for group time at the beginning. Check-In helps to assure that no one "drops a bomb" at the last moment, revealing some terrible news she has been sitting on throughout the session. The structure of Check-In is intended to assist members to exercise greater mastery of and choice about their experience and expression of difficult emotional material. For example, it may be easier for a particular woman to bring up a difficult issue during Check-In when she knows that her time for this initial discussion is limited than it would be for her to bring it up during a more open discussion period. This is another reason for not abandoning the structure.

Along with Check-Out (described later in this chapter), Check-In can provide several therapeutic benefits. Through Check-In and Check-Out, each member talks about her thoughts and feelings at least twice during each group session. For shy or socially awkward members, Check-In and Check-Out provide brief, structured opportunities to practice and experiment with expressing feelings and sharing with the group. It is not unusual for such members to move from speaking exclusively during Check-In and Check-Out to venturing forth in the more complex arena of unstructured group discussion. For a few individuals, the structure of Check-In and Check-Out may continue to provide the primary opportunities for expression. Although therapists should gently invite the input of such members during the unstructured portions of the group, they should also recognize that developing an ability to share at these times may represent a significant development for some individuals. At the same time, therapists may need to politely curtail more vocal members, assuring them that their concerns will be addressed later in the group.

At the beginning of each session, Check-In facilitates the rapid re-establishment of a culture of respect, connection, and sharing and helps both therapists and group members to become attuned to one another rapidly. Check-In provides the group with information regarding the importance of particular themes for discussion that day and special needs of particular members, so that group time and attention may be allocated on that basis. Check-In institutionalizes the expectation that group members set the agenda for the group and that they hear from and respond to one another to do this.

For the therapists, Check-In provides valuable information about both individual issues and more general group themes they can help tie together or bring to group awareness. Even more important, however, is the therapeutic stance implicitly communicated by this structure. Group members are being asked to articulate and communicate their experiences, feelings, and needs. Group members are being encouraged to take responsibility for asking for and getting help. At the same time, group members are being asked to support one another and to attend to the feelings and needs of others. The group is expected to regulate its own activities and resources so that the concerns and needs of all members can be addressed. This involves careful attention both to one's own experience and to that of others. By incorporating these expectations in the regular structure of the group, the therapists' confidence in the group's ability to accomplish these goals is conveyed. This helps to communicate both the seriousness of the issues with which group members are confronted and the belief that the attendant feelings can be expressed and tolerated (or more readily accepted).

During the first few group sessions, Check-In tends to require more intensive management by the cotherapists. After a few sessions, the flow tends to proceed more naturally on its own, often with very little intervention from the therapists.

GROUP DISCUSSION

An overview of the therapeutic style used during the Group Discussion has been presented in chapter 3. More specific information about group therapy facilitation is presented in chapter 5.

To facilitate the rapid development of group cohesiveness and mutual knowledge, we recommend that a number of specific group activities be used during the early weeks of the group. These are described in detail later in this chapter. Over the course of the 16 weeks, the Group Discussion element—which comprises the majority of group time—transitions from relatively structured to a format that is less structured and is based on issues that are introduced by the group members themselves. Later in this chapter, we provide guidance about managing the transition from more structured to less structured discussion. As noted, the intention of the recommended activities is to facilitate the development of mutual knowledge, interconnectedness, and group cohesion and to make certain types of material quickly available for group discussions. Some techniques are also aimed at establishing a broader life context and identity for each member beyond simply having breast cancer. Many breast cancer patients might have a sense that their identity is equated with cancer, and this often limits them from drawing on relevant experiences and coping skills from other areas of their lives.

Many group therapists believe that it is best to allow this sense of connection to develop on its own and to allow the material to emerge organically and spontaneously, without the therapist relying on specific structured techniques. Although this is useful for long-term psychotherapy groups, we have found it to be less valuable for time-limited groups, particularly with medical populations. At the opposite end of the continuum from therapists who advocate no predetermined structure, some therapists believe that it is better to continually structure each group, ensuring that all "important" topics are covered and lessons learned about these topics for patients with a specific medical or psychological diagnosis. We believe that a highly structured approach can be valuable for very short-term groups (8 weeks or less) and those that are aimed primarily at providing information and teaching behavioral skills.

Our experience has shown us that beginning with some structure to the group topics and interactions and then transitioning to a more open structure is optimal for groups of the length described here and with patients facing a life-threatening or life-altering illness (e.g., other types of cancer, cardiac disease). Thus, a degree of initial structure followed by reduced therapist-initiated structure serves to stimulate group cohesion and member participation and to establish the culture of what to discuss and how to discuss it. This helps groups to focus quickly and stay focused on important issues. With too little initial structure, groups require more therapist intervention throughout to maintain therapeutic focus. With too much structure for too long, groups may continue to rely on the therapists for direction and substance.

After the early, structured sessions, Check-In should be used as a springboard for group discussion. Sometimes a clear theme arises from the Check-In of several members. At other times, there may be several disparate issues that appear to be important for different members. In either case, the therapists should not have difficulty finding topics to ask about and members willing to talk about their experiences. When concerns arise that seem likely to stimulate discussion, the therapists should invite and facilitate discussion of these concerns for as long as it appears to be valuable for the group. The therapists should also take responsibility for making sure that the needs of individual members identified during Check-In are met to the extent possible in later discussion. In general, however, therapists should keep in mind that the topics selected for discussion are less important than the process of discussing them. Whereas group members are responsible for selecting topics to be discussed, therapists are responsible for helping patients express their negative as well as positive experiences as authentically as possible. Specific methods for group facilitation are described in chapter 5.

Topic Introduction

Although group members are asked to select topics, therapists can introduce a relevant topic when the discussion stagnates or becomes too superficial and their attempts to stimulate meaningful discussion further are unsuccessful. This should be done with caution, because it may be necessary for group members to struggle through some periods of silence, awkwardness, and anxiety before taking consistent responsibility for initiating and managing their own discussion. However, when it appears to be necessary for the therapists to introduce a topic, one of the following methods may be used:

- asking about a previously unfinished topic that stimulated substantial discussion;
- asking about reactions to *The Breast Cancer Notebook* material reviewed during the week;
- asking a probing question. These questions can be based on previous group material or may relate to a new topic that is likely to be of interest to the group but that has not been previously discussed in depth. These questions might focus on coping with treatment, adjusting to new circumstances, communicating more effectively with others, or dealing with sexuality and intimate relationships. Questions may also relate to more existential issues, such as changes in self-image, values, and goals. (Other topics commonly raised by groups are presented in chapter 5.)

When the group has taken up the discussion, the therapists should again take a back seat and intervene only to facilitate the discussion.

End of Meeting Approaching

About 10 minutes before Check-Out, it is useful for the therapists to announce that the end of the session is approaching. Closing the meeting can sometimes be difficult, especially when emotional issues are being discussed. Letting the group know that 10 minutes remain for discussion can serve to focus the group on essentials and help members begin to summarize important points. It also signals that new "hot" topics should not be pursued in much detail at this time and should be picked up again at the next meeting. Finishing on time is important, because it offers the security of a structure that helps the group to contain unexpected feelings that may arise. Consistent closure also serves to let the group know that whatever occurs in the group, the therapists, although not always active, are nonetheless always in control, maintaining responsibility for holding the frame of the group to keep members safe and secure.

CHECK-OUT

The procedure for Check-Out is similar to the one followed for Check-In. The purpose of Check-Out is to provide each group member with a sense of closure and an opportunity to get what she needs as the session ends. Check-Out is explicitly focused on hearing each member's reaction to the group that day. Going around the room, each group member is asked to speak for 1 or 2 minutes about her experience in the group. Members are encouraged to share their emotional responses with the group and any important or final feelings and thoughts regarding any of the content of the session. Check-Out also provides an opportunity to complete important communications or interactions with specific individuals. Check-Out also allows each member to begin to organize her emotional experience during the session and to continue to reflect on it. Topics for future sessions may also be identified at this time.

Focusing Check-Out specifically on each member's reaction to the group session itself reinforces the importance of the feelings of each member. Check-Out provides the group with important information regarding the response of all group members to particular themes and interactions. This is especially important for the group when very strong emotions have been expressed, conflict between group members has occurred, or concerns raised during the session may have upset a member in some way.

Through Check-Out, members are able to reassure themselves and one another of their ability to withstand the events of that session. Check-Out also provides the group with the opportunity to respond to the needs of any member who is ending the group in a state of distress or conflict. Thus, Check-Out helps members to develop confidence in the ability of the group to function as a container for powerful issues, to tolerate the expression of powerful emotions, and to respond to the experience and needs of each member. Over the course of the sessions, therapists are likely to observe considerable growth in group members' ability to synthesize their emotional reactions to the group discussion, often paired with new perspectives on present or past concerns, new willingness to ask for support both within and outside of the group, and greater tolerance and empathy for the experience and feelings of others.

CLOSING RELAXATION

The most important purpose of the Closing Relaxation exercises is to provide an opportunity for participants to integrate emotions experienced during the group and to reduce arousal related to those emotions. Closing Relaxation also provides an opportunity to practice and teach techniques that participants can use at home, including more elaborate and longer relaxation and imagery techniques. Closing Relaxation is approximately 10 minutes long (see Exhibit 4.2).

A variety of techniques can be used at different sessions, which may include progressive and autogenic muscle relaxation, guided imagery, and meditation techniques. Other types of imagery are sometimes incorporated, such as imagining a part of their lives that participants wish to change as a scene projected into the distance, with an adjacent scene containing an image of how things might be if that aspect of their lives were changed. Participants are then asked to consider what they can begin to do to shift from the current to the desired image. If particularly powerful emotional issues have been raised during the group, reference to them is sometimes incorporated in the closing relaxation, with suggestions to encourage closure now and re-address these issues at future sessions, emphasizing the capacity of each participant to contain these thoughts and feelings comfortably.

Mental imagery may be used, especially at the end of the session, to put into focus some aspect of what transpired. However, suggestions are always nondirective, giving group participants a high degree of per-

---

EXHIBIT 4.2

Sample Closing Relaxation Exercise

The following is an example of a general imagery exercise that might be appropriate for Closing Relaxation.

1. Tense your fists, raise your shoulders, squeeze your eyes, and take a deep breath. Then let go and relax. Imagine your mind relaxing into your breath, and your breath relaxing into your body, and your body relaxing into the chair.
2. As your body continues to relax, imagine yourself in a safe and comfortable place, such as a safe room or a garden, or whatever comes to mind. It may be a place you've been to before or a place you wish you could go to. You can remove any discomfort from this place and add to it anything that will help you feel safe and comfortable.

---

sonal control and choice over the exercise. The goal of the technique is to induce a state of safety, relaxation, and comfort. Imagery might also be used to explore issues of personal meaning to group members; however, it is never used in such a way as to suggest a direct influence on the disease process, such as by imagining immune cells attacking the cancer. There is no evidence that such manipulative imagery helps survival. Independent of survival potential, however, such approaches tend to (a) foster false hope; (b) encourage avoidance of current real issues; (c) promote a view that personal ego is omnipotent, able to wish the cancer away; and (d) result in feelings of personal failure if the cancer progresses. In contrast, focusing on enhancing general skills such as relaxation, emotional management, and the ability to directly confront one's fears and hopes in a calm and relaxed manner assists one in better coping with the cancer and living as fully as one can in each moment.

Following the induction of a state of moderate relaxation, specific exercises can be used to summarize and integrate themes brought up in the group. Several examples are presented below. (Therapists would pick just one to facilitate at any given meeting.)

1. Imagine a scene off in the distance, where
   - you have little control over an aspect of your cancer treatment or your life at present ... (then, after about five breaths) Now imagine a different scene where you have control over some aspect of your cancer treatment or your life at present ... (pause for at least five breaths before ending the exercise)
   - there is some stressor in your life that you feel you don't respond well to ... (then, after about five breaths) Now imagine the same stressor, but now imagine a scenario where you respond optimally in the face of that stressor ... (pause for at least five breaths before ending the exercise)
   - you see yourself the way you used to be, and you can say goodbye to that self ... (then, after about five breaths) Now see yourself the way you are now, and welcome and appreciate the qualities you currently respect in yourself ... (pause for at least five breaths) Now imagine yourself the way you'd like to be 1 year from now. What characteristics would you like to have? (Pause for at least five breaths before ending the exercise.)
2. Now, ready to return to the room, begin noticing that when you inhale you raise your chest. (Begin speaking increasingly louder and faster, until at the end you are speaking in a normal voice.) Breath in a little deeper with the next inhale. With the next inhale or the one after, let your chest and eyes raise way up toward the ceiling. Then refocus in the room feeling clear and focused and full of calm energy to help you through the rest of the day.

Examples of other experiential techniques, including relaxation, meditation, self-hypnosis, and imagery techniques, are provided in chapter 5 and the Appendix.

Use of The Breast Cancer Notebook

Educational material and resources are particularly important for primary breast cancer patients, who are struggling with a new diagnosis and a new disease and whose needs for information may therefore be high. *The Breast Cancer Notebook* is such a resource; it emphasizes personal experience and response to the information presented as much as the information itself. The notebook's primary purpose is to provide an environment and a process through which each group member has the opportunity to assess and reflect on the impact that breast cancer has had on specific areas of her life. It is also intended to provide a focus on prominent areas of concern for women with breast cancer, with the expectation that consideration of these issues will carry over into the group meetings.

The Breast Cancer Notebook is divided into 12 chapters, or topic areas. For each chapter, a brief introduction is provided, followed by a series of questions intended to allow members to personalize the material. For each chapter, members also have the option to pursue the topic in more depth by referring to brochures, books, Web sites, and other resources listed. A more specific description of the contents is provided in chapter 7.

The aim of *The Breast Cancer Notebook* is to provide information in such a way that the coping abilities of members are given gentle and confident support, with the message that, with regard to each topic, each participant can mobilize her internal and external resources in a manner appropriate to her individual circumstances. In this model, the emphasis is not on conveying specific information with the expectation that each member will learn it. Instead, the emphasis is on encouraging each participant to gather as much information as she finds helpful, in an interactive manner, so that she can incorporate the information meaningfully into her recovery process. The focus rests on how each woman wants to use the material in the notebook and, ideally, on fostering her own insight into the effects of her choices and on her ability to move forward to a new psychological homeostasis.

As mentioned in the section earlier in this chapter on the Pregroup Intake Interview, we recommend that each group member be given *The Breast Cancer Notebook* before the group begins. She should be asked to look at the general structure of the notebook and told to feel free to look at any material that is specifically useful to her at the present time. She should be encouraged to review the first chapter, "Finding Your Way," before the group begins.

The sequence of the chapters in *The Breast Cancer Notebook* is keyed to the developmental life of the group over the 16 weeks, and it allows for some flexibility in implementation by the therapists. A very important function of the notebook is to raise key issues in the lives of group members (e.g., family, work, body image) in a way that facilitates and sets a context for their open discussion. This is likely to be particularly important in the context of a time-limited group, where allowing each issue simply to emerge over time might result in critical topics never being addressed.

The cotherapists should not use *The Breast Cancer Notebook* directively. That it, the chapters are not intended to set the topic for that week's discussion; rather, the material suggests possible topics for discussion. If the material is relevant to a particular members' concerns at a particular meeting, it may assist the member and the group by stimulating discussion. Group members should feel free at any session to refer to material from any part of the notebook, not just to material for that particular week. The therapists or the group members should alter the order of reading assignments if necessary to better match what the group is working on. Over time, we expect that the notebook will become an integral and organic part of the group. During the earlier sessions, however, the material may be used to initiate discussions to get the group interacting along common themes.

At the end of each meeting, the cotherapists should describe the chapter in *The Breast Cancer Notebook* that is related to the next meeting. There are 16 group meetings and 12 chapters in the notebook, so a new chapter will not be introduced every week. The therapists may also wish to review the questions at the end of the chapter with the group, particularly during the first few weeks when the group and the notebook are more closely integrated. Before Check-In, the therapists can remind members to bring up any important reactions, thoughts, or feelings they may have about that week's chapter as part of their Check-In (among other things). These issues can be pursued during subsequent discussion as appropriate. Members should be encouraged to share both positive and negative reactions.

When *The Breast Cancer Notebook* describes a specific activity for the next group session, the cotherapists should describe the planned activity during the previous meeting. The therapists should emphasize that each group member has the option not to participate in that activity if she chooses not to do so. (We have never had a group member choose not to participate in one of the activities.) If the activity involves sharing specific types of material with other group members, the therapists should indicate that group members might plan in advance what they want to say, or they may choose to participate spontaneously. The goal is always for each group member to use the notebook and the activities in the way that feels more relevant and helpful to her.

It is important to note that none of the activities described in *The Breast Cancer Notebook* (or described in the sections later in this chapter on specific group meetings) should be viewed as mandatory. The co-therapists may decide that a particular activity does not match the group's needs at a particular time or that the material that might be generated by an activity is already present in the group discussion. In such a case, the therapists might decide to skip or delay a particular recommended activity. Or, the therapists may prefer to substitute another activity with which they are more comfortable to accomplish some of the same objectives. It should be noted that the activities that are suggested for early sessions are described in the notebook, so it may be useful to acknowledge departures from this format so as not to confuse group members.

Structure of Group Discussions Over Time

Throughout the 16 weeks of therapy, each Group Discussion is framed by the structure of Opening Relaxation and Check-In at the beginning and Check Out and Closing Relaxation at the end. The structure and process of the group is different depending on whether the group is in its early, middle, or final meetings. The general structure of meetings is described for each of these phases.

EARLY MEETINGS: INITIAL SUPPORTIVE STRUCTURING

In the context of a short-term therapy group, structured activities aimed at facilitating a rapid process of joining and sharing with others can be extremely useful. The activities incorporated into the first few sessions are intended to facilitate the rapid development of a group culture, a culture that says, "We can talk about this here." In addition, these activities assist each group member in telling others her particular story regarding breast cancer, its impact on her life, and about who she was and is before and apart from her disease. As a part of this process, these activities assist in facilitating awareness and acknowledgment of the uniqueness and individuality of each group member, her circumstances, and her experience. This is viewed as a precondition for authentic rapport.

Structuring the First Session

The first session is the only one that does not begin with Opening Relaxation and Check-In, because members obviously do not know what to expect at this point. The cotherapists should begin by welcoming members and briefly introducing themselves (e.g., name, professional role and background, interest in present project). Indicating that there will be more opportunity later in the session to talk in more depth, the therapists should ask the women in the group simply to go around the room and tell others their names and anything else that they would consider important to say as part of an initial introduction. These initial introductions should be limited to about 1 minute per group member.

Next, the cotherapists should describe the purpose of the group and the role they will play in it. In general, the therapists should indicate that the group is a place where members can discuss personal concerns. Group members should be told that the therapists are there to assist group members in discussing specific personal concerns, help them to feel safe expressing their feelings about what is transpiring in their lives, search for ways to cope with their treatment and its consequences, and learn to adjust to what is occurring in a way that will help them to live each day as fully as possible. Therapists must remember that people from all walks of life and various ways of viewing the world come together in this (for them) unusual setting. They want to know how the group functions, in terms of what is discussed as well as how issues raised are to be discussed. The initial meeting is an important first step in forming the group culture that is to continue in future meetings.

Next, it is useful for the therapists to discuss the guidelines for the group frame described earlier in this chapter (time, attendance, confidentiality, socializing). It is also helpful to provide information about the structure of each meeting and the nature and purpose of Opening Relaxation, Check-In, Check-Out, and Closing Relaxation.

In addition, we have found that it is useful to provide an activity that fosters the expectation that group members will talk, listen, and provide support to others and that provides some basis for interpersonal connections and shared experience. At the first session, group members bring with them not only their hopes but also anxiety and fears about joining the group. Facilitating the expression of these feelings permits group members to be more available to other experiences. For many members, however, expressing such private feelings publicly to the entire group may be initially too threatening.

A simple exercise works well for this purpose (see Table 4.2). The cotherapists ask each group member to pair with one other woman in the group. Pairs can simply be assigned by going around the room. If there is an odd number of group members, a triad can be formed or the

TABLE 4.2

First Session Culture Building Exercise

Minutes	Activity
0–2	Tricia tells Nancy about concerns and negative expectations regarding the group.
	Nancy listens without comment.
2–3	Nancy tells Tricia a summary of what she has heard.
3–5	Nancy tells Tricia about concerns and negative expectations regarding the group.
	Tricia listens without comment.
5–6	Tricia tells Nancy a summary of what she has heard.
6–12	Regroup for brief group discussion of experience: Similarities? Differences? Surprises?
	Choose new pairs.
12–14	Tricia tells Cheryl about hopes and positive expectations regarding the group.
	Cheryl listens without comment.
14–15	Cheryl tells Tricia a summary of what she has heard.
15–17	Cheryl tells Tricia about hopes and positive expectations about the group.
	Tricia listens without comment.
17–18	Tricia tells Cheryl a summary of what she has heard.
18–25	Regroup for brief group discussion of experience: Similarities? Differences? Surprises? How are you feeling now?

Note. Tricia, Nancy, and Cheryl are fictitious group members used as examples.

female therapist can ask one of the members to do the activity with her. Each woman is asked to speak to the other for 2 minutes about her concerns, worries, apprehensions, and negative expectations about the group. We have found that it is helpful to allow group members to talk about their concerns first. This tends to help them to be more receptive to the positive expectations in themselves and others that follow in the next segment.

While the first woman is talking about her expectations, the second woman simply listens for a 2-minute period. After that, the woman who listened is asked to spend 1 minute telling the woman who spoke what she has heard and understood, without in any way offering advice or countering or interpreting what has been said. The explicit task is simply to reflect in one's own words the experience that has been shared by the other person. This process is then repeated with reversed roles. One therapist serves as a time-keeper during this process to keep the dyads moving along. Part of the benefit of this exercise is the initial safety that comes with the brevity of the exercise and structured interaction. The group is then asked to re-form, and members are invited to share with others anything they wish to share about this experience.

Following a brief group discussion, members are asked to pair with a new partner, for example, the woman to her other side, and to repeat this process, this time sharing and reflecting and spending 2 minutes talking about her positive hopes and expectations. This is again followed by brief group discussion. Using this exercise, we have found that at Check-Out, anxiety is lower and that positive anticipation (some guarded, some enthusiastic) is expressed. Group members tend to leave the first meeting in animated conversations with one another, rather than in silent isolation.

Next, the cotherapists should spend a few minutes describing *The Breast Cancer Notebook*, how it will be used during the group, and how group members might use it outside the group. It should be emphasized that the questions at the end of each chapter are for group members' own use only and that women will not be asked to turn in their answers or to share them with other group members unless they specifically wish to do so. The therapists should then invite any thoughts, comments, feelings, or reactions in response to chapter 1, "Finding Your Way," and facilitate a discussion of these reactions.

As the end of the session approaches, the therapists should announce this and then should introduce chapter 2 from *The Breast Cancer Notebook*, "How Are You Coping With Breast Cancer?" The therapists should explain that over the next 2 weeks the group will be taking the time to find out about each woman's personal story, about her experience with breast cancer, and to learn more about her as a person. About half the group members will have a chance to talk about their personal experience during the second week, and the other half will have a chance to do so during the following week.

Next, the therapists should briefly remind group members of the purpose and structure of Check-Out. Going around the room from a point indicated by one of the therapists, each woman should take 1 to 2 minutes to reflect about her experience of the group that evening. Some of the things that the women might consider addressing during this time include the following: Did the group meet her expectations? Was anything surprising? Was it harder or easier than she expected? How is she feeling about the other group members? About the therapists? About being in the group?

Finally, the group should end with a simple 5-minute closing relaxation, perhaps focusing on calming the mind and attending to the breath. (It is best to start with simpler techniques and introduce more complex relaxation techniques later as members acquire more experience.) This will assist each group member in leaving the group feeling comfortable, irrespective of what was aroused during the session.

Table 4.3 provides an outline of the activities during the first group meeting.

The Second and Third Sessions

The second and third sessions begin to follow what will become the customs of the group. The cotherapists should begin the session within a few minutes of the starting time by getting up and closing the door as a way of announcing that it is time to begin. The therapists should remind group members of planned absences and give them any information they may have about absent members. They can also ask if anyone has information about anyone else who is missing unexpectedly.

Opening Relaxation

A simple relaxation exercise should be conducted, focusing on calming the body and mind. (It is useful to alternate leading the relaxation be-

---

TABLE 4.3

Outline of Activities During the First Group Meeting

Topic	Duration (*approximate*)
1. Introduction of therapists	4 minutes
2. Initial brief (1 minute) introduction of group members	15 minutes
3. Description of nature and purpose of group, role of therapists	5 minutes
4. Discussion of guidelines regarding the group frame ▪ Dates, length of group ▪ Starting and ending times ▪ Attendance issues (attending each group, notifying of absence) ▪ Confidentiality ▪ Socializing	10 minutes
5. Description of structure within group meetings ▪ Check-In and Check-Out ▪ Opening and Closing Relaxation	5 minutes
6. Culture building exercise and discussion	25 minutes
7. Description of *Breast Cancer Notebook* and its use during group	5 minutes
8. Discuss reactions to first chapter, "Finding Your Way"	30 minutes
9. Introduction of second chapter, "Breast Cancer Treatment"	3 minutes
10. Description of focus for second and third sessions (stories from group members)	3 minutes
11. Check-Out	10 minutes
12. Closing Relaxation	5 minutes

tween cotherapists.) The therapist who is not leading the relaxation can watch for late-comers and motion them to sit quietly.

Check-In

Next, the group should be reminded briefly about the purpose of Check-In. They should be reminded that, among other things, it may be helpful to mention their reactions to this week's chapter from *The Breast Cancer Notebook*. Beginning with a starting point indicated by the therapists, women should take turns and check in for 1 to 2 minutes each. It may be necessary initially to prompt individual members regarding the types of things that might be mentioned during Check-In. As indicated above, if members begin to get into extended discussions of issues during Check-In, they can be reminded that the group can come back to these issues a bit later.

Beginning with the second session, the therapists should remain flexible about structured exercises or guided discussions. That is, if a particular member is in crisis or group discussion about a particular topic appears to be more important at the moment than the planned exercise, the exercise should be more limited in time or postponed until the following week. Such changes in plans should be made explicit, and it is generally helpful to present them as a choice to the group.

Personal Stories

Provided that there are no immediate crises or other critical issues, the cotherapists should remind the group that over the next 2 weeks the group will hear each woman's story about her experience with breast cancer. This may include how she was diagnosed, the nature of her cancer, her treatment, what she is still undergoing or struggling with, her reactions, and how her life has been affected. The therapists should indicate that this should take about 5 to 8 minutes per member, with some opportunity for the group to ask questions to help them understand each woman's situation. During both the second and third session, about half the women in the group should tell their stories. It seems best to allow group members to proceed in any order they choose. It may be helpful for some women to have a chance to talk about this right away, whereas others may prefer to wait until after they have heard from a few other members.

Members who are telling their stories can be gently prompted by the therapists if necessary. However, it is important to remember that these should be the women's own stories, told in whatever manner feels most helpful to them and communicating the information that they feel is most important for the group to know. After each story, the therapists and group members should have an opportunity to ask clarifying questions or offer personal reactions for a minute or two. Women should not be pressured to talk about areas that they do not feel comfortable discussing. The therapists should respect and honor each woman's experience, thereby setting the tone for the group, and should thank each woman for sharing her experience.

Each week, after half the women in the group have had an opportunity to tell their stories, the therapists should facilitate a general discussion about what the group has learned, group members' reactions to other members, and other themes and issues that have been raised.

Winding Down

About 10 minutes before the end of the open discussion, the cotherapists should announce the approaching end of the discussion and that the group will have an opportunity to continue with these issues during the following session. The session should end with Check-Out, focusing on each group member's reactions to the session, followed by Closing Relaxation.

Before members leave at the end of the second session, the therapists should announce that the chapter from *The Breast Cancer Notebook* for the following week is chapter 3, "Breast Cancer Treatment." At the end of the third session, the cotherapists should announce that the next chapter (chapter 4) is "Coping With Treatment Side Effects." Depending on the specific composition of the group, the therapists may want to acknowledge that some portions of these chapters may not seem immediately relevant for women who have finished treatment but that they still provide a useful opportunity to reflect on their experience with the treatment.

(See Table 4.1 for a timetable for Groups 2–16. Groups 2 and 3 differ from the others only in that the general discussion focuses on the women telling their personal stories.)

The Fourth Session

If the group has been structured as described for the first three weeks, a great deal of information would have been introduced about each woman's experience with cancer and treatment. We have found that it is helpful to allow a more open discussion during the fourth week so that members have an opportunity to respond to and discuss this material and how it makes them feel about being in the group. In addition, the chapters that have been reviewed from *The Breast Cancer Notebook* about breast cancer and its treatment may raise issues, and would be useful to allow time for that discussion. Therefore, we recommend that the fourth session be used as an opportunity for this general discussion, facilitated by the cotherapists. This means that the fourth session follows a more typical group format, as outlined in Table 4.1.

After Check-Out and before Closing Relaxation, the therapists should introduce the next chapter from *The Breast Cancer Notebook*, "Communicating With Members of Your Medical Team" (chapter 5).

Additional Structured Activities for the Fifth and Sixth Group Meetings

The cotherapists may decide at this point to begin eliciting expressions of concerns from the group and approach group meetings in a more unstructured fashion (as we have recommended for Session 4). However, we have found that providing two more structured sessions may be of significant benefit. The two sessions described below can help group members learn to express themselves more openly, resulting in a feeling of self-worth, appreciation of other's worth, and a close bonding of group members. This lays a strong foundation for the rest of the group. However, if the therapists determine that open discussion or alternative activities would be more useful at this point than the structured activities proposed, the recommended activities should not be viewed as mandatory.

As noted, there is plenty of material for the group to discuss by the fourth group meeting. At the same time, most of the material included during these first weeks had focused on the cancer rather than on the woman with cancer. This is deliberate. It is our experience that group members tend to have a strong need to talk about their experiences with breast cancer first and to connect with one another around these experiences. However, we have also found that, over time, an obstacle to the development of a sense of group cohesiveness and interconnectedness is that, with the exception of their shared status as breast cancer patients, group members know virtually nothing about one another as women. It can be difficult for group members to risk expressing their thoughts and feelings about the deeply held and personal issues that their cancer experience has touched on without having a sense of being perceived, known, and understood by others in a fuller way. For this reason, discussions may be intellectual, abstract, and disconnected from immediate experience.

The activities described below for the fifth and sixth sessions focus on the person who has cancer, rather than the disease, its treatments, and the medical environments they involve. These activities are intended to facilitate the process of each group member presenting herself more fully to the group, and thereby gaining a deeper, broader, and more authentic connection with other group members.

The activity for the fifth meeting should be described to group members at the end of the fourth group meeting, after Check-Out and before Closing Relaxation, after chapter 5 of *The Breast Cancer Notebook* ("Communicating With Members of Your Medical Team") is introduced. This will help each member to prepare for the activity in any way she wishes. Each member is encouraged to bring a photograph of herself between ages 5 and 12 to the fifth meeting. Each member will be asked to talk for about 5 minutes about her life and identity before breast cancer based on where she comes from and her family of origin. The therapists should describe a variety of areas that group members may wish to touch on, emphasizing their early family life, adolescence, early relationships, identity, and aspirations. Members may wish to share both positive and negative events. Therapists should explicitly mention that group members may wish to talk about cancer-related bereavements (e.g., death of mother or close relative) if this occurred in their early lives. Obviously, it is not possible to cover all areas in the available time, so each member must choose the events that she considers most important for others to know about her. Members may plan in advance what they want to say if this is helpful, or they may choose to participate spontaneously. Members should be given the option of not participating in this exercise if they do not feel comfortable with it, but we have never had a member choose not to do so.

The Fifth Session

Provided that there are no urgent issues for the group to discuss and following Opening Relaxation and Check-In, the therapists should proceed with the activity as planned, allowing about 5 minutes per member.

As each group member talks about herself, the childhood photograph is passed among the other members. After each member speaks, 2 to 3 minutes are allocated for other group members to talk about their own responses to the story they have heard. This exercise provides a powerful and often very emotional introduction, as the presentations begin to fill in the identities of other group members and to change them from strangers to differentiated fellow travelers worthy of respect and understanding. Members begin to feel perceived and understood by others. For the therapists, this exercise provides valuable historical and psychological information about group members and helps both therapists and other group members to understand each woman's individual responses and ways of coping.

The remaining time in the session should be allocated to general discussion of issues. This exercise is typically very stimulating for members, so there should be a good deal to discuss. This is followed by Check-Out, according to the usual structure.

After Check-Out and before Closing Relaxation, the therapists should introduce chapter 6 of *The Breast Cancer Notebook*, "Family and Friends." They should acknowledge that the notebook is now switching gears somewhat, moving from a focus on the disease itself to a broader look at the impact of breast cancer on other important areas of group members' lives. One purpose of focusing on this area is to help the women in the group explore their lives more fully. Group members are obviously more than their breast cancer, and exploring their full personas in the group helps them and other members.

If the cotherapists believe that this activity is not in synch with the group's priorities or that enough of this material has been or can be accessed without the activity, the activity should be viewed as optional. If the activity is planned, the therapists should indicate that the next group session will be the second devoted to issues related to family. This discussion will shift during the next week from family of origin to current family, and in particular it will focus on family issues with which group members are currently struggling. This should be introduced in such a way that the experiences of all group members are respected and can be included. For example, women without partners or children in the group may wish to let the group know about who is important in their lives ("chosen family") and their struggles with the relationships they currently have and those they may wish they had. The cotherapists should indicate that some of the questions in chapter 6 of *The Breast Cancer Notebook* may be helpful to members as they think about these issues.

The description of this activity should be followed by Closing Relaxation.

The Sixth Session

If the activity is used, the sixth session should be structured in much the same way as the fifth, with members participating in the exercise and guided discussion as planned. As before, if Check-In reveals a significant crisis or other important issue to attend to, the exercise can be modified or postponed. Each member is asked to spend about 5 minutes, first setting a context by talking about her family and then talking about what she is struggling with currently in relation to her family or in relation to other important relationships. Again, it is important for the therapists to communicate respect for each woman's situation and perspective. A member should tell other group members enough information about who is in her family and what her relationship is like with these people that the group has a context for understanding her concerns. However, the emphasis here should be on family issues or other important relationships with which members are currently struggling.

Unless this discussion is correctly managed by the therapists, it could turn into a comparison of the quality of members' families and support networks that could hamper some members' abilities to discuss their own concerns (e.g., about not having a family or partner). With skillful management, however, group members will have a rich and deep base of knowledge about one another as a basis for interconnection and authentic communication by the end of the sixth session.

MIDDLE MEETINGS: TRANSITIONING TO LESS STRUCTURE

Although the structure of Opening Relaxation, Check-In, Check-Out, and Closing Relaxation is retained throughout the life of the group, by the seventh session there should be little need for the therapists to provide structured activities or structured discussion directly based on *The Breast Cancer Notebook*. Rather, the material can be used in a more general, indirect way. For example, the therapists can ask whether the assigned chapter stimulated any thought in relation to a particular discussion. By this time, the group agenda is generally overflowing and group members are ready to take over and talk.

During the next few sessions, however, some difficulty frequently emerges as the group assumes responsibility for the structure and content of most of the group time. Much depends on the way earlier meetings proceeded. Unless the therapists have been careful to support the group members in taking responsibility for the sessions despite the degree of structure provided, transition to member-initiated discussion may be difficult. The more therapists have elicited topics of concern among group members, the easier the transition to members taking the lead in discussion. There is no simple formula for deciding the extent to which therapists need to be active. Some groups are very active in initiating important topics to discuss in meaningful ways such that the therapists need not be as active. Other groups may be slower to initiate topics of concern to them or may tend to explore topics that appear to be less relevant, such that therapists must structure the groups to a greater extent. In these cases, the early, more structured sessions may be viewed as laying a foundation for independence in later sessions as long as the therapists have kept this eventual "weaning" in mind.

The therapists should be understanding and forthcoming about the importance of making the transition from a structured discussion to group selection of topics that it considers most important, and the challenge this transition creates for the group. Therapists need to stress the importance of group members deciding the content to be discussed that is most meaningful for them. The challenge to the group parallels the challenge in individual members' lives—to create a sense of meaning and connection in an uncertain and impermanent context. All in all, any difficulty in transitioning to fuller group self-reliance is more than made up for by the level of connection, trust, and intimacy developed during the first few group sessions. Therapists can reinforce the notion that group members have the most to gain from one another, not from the therapists. Sometimes, a group will generate on its own a list of topics members would like to cover. This may be helpful to the group, but the therapists should also remind the group that it should remain flexible enough to be responsive during each session to the material generated during Check-In and to the changing needs of each member.

Some degree of difficulty is a natural part of this developmental process. It is important that the therapists not respond to the pressure to provide group members by "entertaining" or otherwise attempt to interject their own experiences to make the group more "exciting." During this period, groups may struggle with issues related to establishing norms, leadership, and a space for all members. Some group members may hesitate to ask the group for the things they need or fear being seen as taking on a leadership role in the group. Although at times there may be a hesitancy to discuss issues important to the members, at other times there may be several topics arising in quick succession that need to be addressed. Group members may express diverging points of view about which they feel passionately (e.g., religion and spirituality, complementary medicine). Interpersonal conflicts may emerge at this point around the agenda of the group. It is important for the therapists to help the group navigate these, allowing the respectful expression of each group member's needs and opinions.

FINAL MEETINGS: TERMINATION

The final meetings of the group should focus increasingly on group termination. It is important that group termination be approached consciously and thoughtfully by the therapists. In fact, the group's time-limited nature should be kept in mind throughout the therapy duration. The final sessions may be difficult for many members. Bonds that have been formed will be coming to a close, with associated feelings of loss. Discussion in these final meetings can focus on finding social support in their lives, as well as what the group has meant to them. In keeping with promoting active coping, it is useful to ask how the group member intends to continue developing in the way that she has begun in the group. It is also important to allow for sadness and loss to be discussed. Grieving about the loss of the group may help to prepare members for grieving about other aspects of their lives. The therapists may suggest follow-ups to other groups, activities, or therapy, as desired by each individual member.

Although we believe that group termination is useful for women with a first occurrence of breast cancer, we realize that women with recurrent or metastatic breast cancer often benefit from continued group participation, because they face new stressors and circumstances on a daily basis.

Group members often spontaneously broach the subject of termination by making reference to the value of the group, their mixed feelings at its ending, their future relationships with each other, and their plans after the group has ended. Such expressions should be supported by the therapists, without allowing the group to use premature or artificial closure as a way to avoid either additional work that may still be accomplished in the time remaining or wallowing in sadness at the group ending. If discussion of the group ending does not arise spontaneously, the therapists should raise it, initially simply by pointing out that there are only a certain number of weeks remaining in the life of the group.

The group may change during these final meetings in several ways. Sometimes group members may begin to feel "better" and have a tendency to keep the discussion lighter in nature and focus on positive plans for the future. Some of this is valuable. It makes little sense to delve into new emotional territory during the final minutes of the last session. It is equally important, however, not to allow discussion to become overly shallow or future-oriented when there are still several sessions remaining. If the group seems headed in this direction, it can be useful for the therapist to note that the mood of the group seems to have changed. If necessary, the therapist may ask group members whether they believe this is related to the approaching end of the group or about what still may be valuable to discuss during the time remaining.

Occasionally, therapists may encounter feelings about ending the group that are externalized onto some other event or person. For example, distress in ending the group may arise in discussions of a new hoped-for cancer treatment that did not pan out or in a member hearing that a friend has just died of cancer. Therapists should be cautious about stating such interpretations, which would have dubious benefits for the group members at that point and only serve to portray the therapist as the group's "analyst." Instead, therapists can ask directly about group members' feelings and explore these feelings in personal and specific terms. Doing so assists group members in examining what may underlie their feelings at the moment.

Feelings of helplessness often arise toward the end of group therapy. This may be especially true of group members who have recently finished oncotherapy. These members have the double impact of ending two therapies that may have helped to manage anxieties regarding future health and quality of life. Others who became anxious when they ended treatment prior to the group forming may experience renewed anxiety. Still others may have rejoiced at termination of the oncotherapy, which they experienced as eroding their quality of life, but now become anxious at the prospect of ending a therapy they experienced as supporting their quality of life. Therapists must be on the lookout for such reactions and attempt to address them directly. The ability to end this therapy with both appreciation and regret will assist group members to move on with the next phase of their recovery and with their lives.

Members may express a wide range of plans for contact with each other and for seeking future therapeutic support after the group has ended. This variation may range from a desire for a great deal of contact with other group members to no particular desire for contact, from specific plans to seek additional therapy to no plans at all. Members' assessment of the value of the group is likely to range from enthusiastic endorsement to reservation of judgment to disappointment at how little of the potential of the group was realized. The therapists should endorse any conscious attempt to negotiate termination and any honest expression of feelings about the group, positive or negative, because this will aid in each member's ability to bring closure for herself.

Occasionally, members in a group will make plans to keep the group going without the therapists. (Therapists should be clear that continuing with the therapists is not an option, with the exception of groups of people with recurrent cancer.) The therapists may even believe that some members may indeed benefit from a new group or by continuing the current group. Yet, for people recovering from a first occurrence cancer, it is also important to allow things to end. Moving beyond a self-identity as a cancer patient is important. Therapists must ask themselves, and group members, to what extent this refusal to allow the group to end is simply a refusal to allow a full transition to occur in members' lives. Members' lives have changed, and the extent to which they allow the group to end may be a useful metaphor for allowing the past to give way to their future—a future that can be lived more fully by letting go of the past.

Cotherapist Debriefing

As mentioned, debriefing by the cotherapists following each group meeting is an essential part of the group process. Debriefing among therapists should also consider the interaction between each therapist and the group, as well as between the therapists.

After each group, therapists should take time to review a number factors related to the group:

1. The topics discussed in the group (e.g., lack of control, changes in self-image).
2. The quality of group discussion (e.g., degree of affect, tendency to seek information)
3. Each group member's participation (concerns and quality of expression). For example, "Sally was atypically quiet. Might it be due to her ending treatment?"
4. Things to keep in mind for future sessions. For example, "Next session, if Sally is still distant, let's look for an opportunity to ask her how she is doing, especially now that treatment has ended." Or, "The group has not discussed sexuality at all, and there are only four sessions left. Let's look for opportunity to focus on this, or to bring it up directly if necessary."

Debriefing among cotherapists should also consider the interaction between each therapist and the group, as well as between the cotherapists:

5. How each therapist felt about the group as a whole. For example, did the therapist feel the group was dealing with critical issues, avoiding feelings, or being passive? What were the therapist's reactions and feelings about this?
6. How each therapist felt about his or her activity in the group as a whole. For example, "I seemed to be a little too active this session, trying to help too much." Or, "I need to be less defensive with Joanne. I feel like she challenges me."
7. Each therapist's emotional experience. For example, "I got so sad when Maureen was talking about her daughter."
8. How each therapist felt in his or her relationship to the other therapist. For example, "I was annoyed with you because I felt like you cut Maureen off too soon." Or, "I felt that I jumped in too quickly to 'help' you with Jean."

In assessing the session, cotherapists tend to be better than one therapist at reflecting on the current interaction of the group and planning to be sensitive to particular issues for the upcoming group. If one therapist is facilitating the group alone, this self-evaluation is equally important and should be made a formal part of each group.

Suggestions for debriefing (and suggested forms for self-debriefing) are included in the Appendix.

Group Psychotherapy Facilitation 5

This chapter describes specific intervention techniques as well as therapeutic principles meant to serve as general guidelines. By and large, what follows constitutes the majority of what therapists do in this therapeutic approach. The context provided in earlier chapters prepares for this material. The material presented in this chapter should be considered the "heart" of the therapy; in our experience, when used as described, it results in the maximum benefit for patients. We assume that therapists have a background in psychotherapy, including active listening, interpersonal therapy, cognitive therapy, existential therapy, and group process. What follows is not meant to be an introduction to and training of these approaches but rather the way these techniques can be used most effectively in this particular setting.

Specific Intervention: Facilitating Group Discussion

Most of the therapeutic interventions used in this approach to group treatment take the form of leading questions asked by the therapists. In general, it is important to ask questions rather than give advice. The therapists attempt to be peripheral to the group discussion, emerging when necessary to help the group stay "on track" or to help specific members explore their concerns. Once members are "doing their work," however, therapists withdraw to the periphery once again. Thus, therapists must appreciate that the group is the most valuable therapist.

EMPATHIC EMPHASIS

Before asking a leading question, it is usually a good idea to make one or more rapport statements. Therapists who rephrase or summarize group members' feelings and topics should make sure they understand what has been said and increase the group members' confidence that they truly do understand members' concerns. Furthermore, members are more likely to follow a therapist's lead if they believe the therapist has been following their feelings and thoughts.

Rapport is best established by therapists listening attentively to patients' expressions and interactions, without making verbal statements as long as the patient is expressing herself authentically (see below) and the group is interacting in a supportive way. Only after acknowledging the feeling and content of an expression or of the discussion as a whole should the therapist attempt to alter the course or quality of the discussion. From time to time, however, no response may be forthcoming from the group, or a response may draw away from a statement worthy of exploration or continuation. In such cases, therapists should reinforce the discussion through a simple and focused rapport statement (see Exhibit 5.1).

When a group member or the group as a whole begins drifting from meaningful expression, the therapist should make a rapport statement, demonstrating an understanding of the feeling and content present in

---

EXHIBIT 5.1

Examples of Rapport Statements

Abbey: I've just found out that the new chemotherapy I've been put on doesn't seem to be shrinking the tumor as much as they'd hoped.

* * *

[If no response from the group is forthcoming]

Therapist: That's really bad news, that the treatment isn't what you had hoped for. You must be disappointed.

* * *

[If response from the group is forthcoming]

Pam: You know, I just read about a new procedure for getting the chemo directly to the cancer cells. It's only for lymphoma patients now, but hopefully they'll get it for us soon.

Therapist: Everyone hopes that a better treatment for cancer will come around, and soon. But Abbey, you must be really disappointed that the treatment you were on isn't working for you now.

---

the discussion and then ask a question to get the group back on track. Redirecting statements can be directed toward a single person (e.g., "Sally, you seem to be worried about the test you took yesterday") or the group in general (e.g., "There seems to be a lot of interest in the group today about new testing procedures").

Again, when the discussion is "going well," therapists are not required to do anything at all, or they may occasionally offer a light "nudge" with a simple rapport statement including both the content and feeling of a discussion. Yet when the quality of expression begins to focus on people or topics outside the group or on general issues of an intellectual nature or when interaction is lacking, therapists should lead the discussion to a more meaningful exchange.

LEADING QUESTIONS

After an empathic base is formed, therapists can ask a few simple open-ended questions to help members express their concerns in a personal, specific, affective manner; this form of questioning can assist in accessing more authentic intimate personal feelings and in exploring other ways of coping with a problem. Staying intellectual about some general impersonal issue is a defense against intimate concerns that threaten to elicit negative affect. Therapists should appreciate some defensive "rebounding" from feeling overwhelmed by events. Yet therapists also must ensure that they (a) do not reinforce defensive avoidance of this kind and (b) gently lead patients back to authentic exploration of their intimate concerns.

Figure 5.1 provides examples of leading questions that facilitate authentic expression and further exploration of concerns. They are organized by the subject and object of the group member's concern, their affect and approach to coping with a problem, adjusting to their new situation, and the style of interaction in which she engages.

Questions can be used to lead to authentic expression (personal, specific, affective leads) and to explore ways to improve living with cancer (active coping, interpersonally relating, and adjusting to current circumstances to live fully in the moment). Authentic expression should be achieved before beginning to explore alternatives.

Personalizing the Subject

When a group member's expression is focused on a subject other than herself, the therapist should ask the group member a question to help her to phrase her concern in more personal terms (see Exhibit 5.2). In general, when the group member is talking about someone or something else, the therapist should ask how the matter affects her personally. For example, if a member says, "My doctor simply is not interested

FIGURE 5.1

Facilitating Group Therapy Discussion

Lead:	Quality of Expression From Inauthentic	Therapeutic Leads To Authentic
1. Subject:	Impersonal–external ⟶	Personal–internal
	(How does that affect you personally?)	
2. Context:	Abstract–general ⟶	Concrete–specific
	(Can you give a specific example of that problem?)	
3. Affect:	Intellectual–repressed ⟶	Emotional expression
	(How did you feel when that happened?)	
4. Coping:	Passive–helpless ⟶	Active–appropriate control
	(What can you do to handle the situation in a way that works better for you?)	
5. Adjustment:	Fixed assumption ⟶	Consider alternatives
	(What would you do if there was nothing more the doctors could do for your cancer?)	
6. Relationship:	Solipsistic–isolated ⟶	Supportive–interactive
	(Has anyone else in the group had that type of experience?)	

Note. Responses are shown on a continuum from the inauthentic (left) to the authentic (right). Therapist leading questions are in parentheses below the arrow. In Items 1–3, the focus is on expression; in Items 4–6, the focus is on exploration. When needed, therapists ask open-ended questions to elicit more authentic member expression. For example, in response to *"Doctors never care what's going on with you, only what's going on with the tumor!"* the therapist might ask one or several of the questions shown in the figure, depending on group members' subsequent responses. From "Existential Group Psychotherapy for Women With Advanced Breast Cancer," by J. Spira, in *Group Psychotherapy for Medically Ill Patients* (p. 197), edited by J. Spira, 1997b, New York: Guilford Press. Copyright 1997 by Guilford Press. Adapted by permission.

in listening to what options his patients might want. He's pretty sure of himself," the therapist can offer a rapport statement ("You seem to be upset with the way your doctor is talking to you") and then ask, "How does it affect you when you are speaking with him and want him to listen to your concerns, but he doesn't?"

This same approach should be used when the group begins focusing on the latest treatments or research in breast cancer. Discussion of these developments does not maximize the benefits of the group. It is more valuable to ask questions that lead group members to examine how this affects them personally. One example might be, "There is obviously a

EXHIBIT 5.2

Personalizing Leads

Sarah: Ever since my mastectomy, Jerry hasn't seemed interested in sex. He still cuddles and is there for me, but that's about it.

Therapist: You seem disappointed that your intimacy has disappeared. How would you like things to be?

---

great deal of interest in the group today about these new treatments. What does this mean for you personally? Will you ask your doctor about it, and if you are ineligible for this approach, how will you feel?"

Specifying the Context

When the context of a member's expression is vague or abstract, the therapist should ask a question that leads the member to phrase her concerns in terms that are more specific and concrete (see Exhibit 5.3). In general, when the member is speaking abstractly or vaguely, without reference to specific time and place, the therapist should ask for a very specific example of how she has experienced this situation. For example, if a group member says, "Doctors are really not interested in listening to what options patients want. They are trained to tell, not to listen," the therapist can offer a rapport statement (e.g., "You don't feel doctors listen to what patients say . . ."), followed by asking, "Has this happened to you? Can you give us an example of an interaction with your doctor when he did not listen to your concerns?" If the group member can generate no specific experiences and the topic seems useful to the group, the therapist can redirect this question to the group, asking about the personal experiences of other group members related to this topic. If no specific experiences are forthcoming, then the topic is not of real concern and it is best to move on.

Speaking in generalities can be seductive. Often patients or the group as a whole can focus on some seemingly important principle with which therapists also agree. Discussions often turn toward lack of psychosocial concern among oncologists, or cancer treatments in general, or to the cutting of cancer research funds or state benefits. A patient might talk about how it is important to relax and let the pain go during radiation treatment or how it is important to let go of old self-images and move to develop a new self-image. However interesting these topics seem, they have limited value if kept in the abstract. Therapists should move rapidly to ask for specific examples of how the patient making these statements has experienced this in her life. Try to elicit as specific

EXHIBIT 5.3

Specifying Leads

Marge was talking about how she felt "wiped out" from her radiation treatment, had low energy, and was sick all the time, and she complained about how she "couldn't do anything else" anymore. Pat, who always had something "wise" to say, offered this:

> *Pat:* Whenever we feel sick from treatment, we just have to tell ourselves that dwelling on it makes it worse, and we just have to force ourselves to focus on what we need to do to get through the day.

> *Therapist:* That sounds like good advice, Pat. The more we focus on something, the more we enhance it. But so we can better understand exactly what you are recommending, can you give a specific example from your own personal experience of a specific time that you've taken this advice and used it?

a story (particular time and place events) where these concerns were experienced. A concrete personal story has far more impact on a patient and the group than an abstract philosophical discussion.

Tolerating Negative Affect

When the expression is personal and specific and of obvious concern to the group member but is stated intellectually or in a way that seems lacking in emotion, the therapist should probe her emotional state. In general, when a member is talking about a difficult subject in emotionally neutral or even overly positive terms, the therapist should ask her what negative feelings that brings up for her. For instance, if a group member is talking somewhat neutrally or even mildly jokingly about the lack of understanding her oncologist has of her condition, the therapist might begin with a rapport statement followed by a prompt to explore the affect: "Here you are, in the midst of a life-threatening illness and debilitating treatment, and you don't feel connected to the person you are counting on to save your life. What kinds of feelings does that bring up in you?"

Avoiding discussing strong feelings that members obviously must have is also common in cancer groups. Sometimes such incongruity takes on absurd proportions. For example, suppose a member with recurrent breast cancer says, "I know exactly how I am going to end my life, once it is clear that there is no more hope. I am going to fly to the Caribbean, get a hotel room with a view of the ocean, and take an overdose of sleeping pills. I have it all planned out. I've gotten the brochures, decided on the hotel, and even checked out their room service menu!" If this is said in an intellectual fashion, void of emotion or even with a hint of wry humor, as if in casual conversation, the therapist might make a rapport statement (e.g., "You obviously have been considering this very important issue for quite a while") and then continue, "This is a very major step you are considering. And you seem to be talking about it so lightly. But when you think about getting sicker, there being no hope, and taking your own life, doesn't that bring up a lot of feelings in you?"

One of the most difficult aspects of group psychotherapy for women with breast cancer is allowing group members to feel negative emotions. (This can be difficult for the therapists as well! After all, didn't we go into psychotherapy to help others feel better?) The importance of allowing these authentic feelings to be experienced by the member cannot be overemphasized. The more a member is allowed to recognize, experience, and express such distressing feelings, the easier it is for her to let them go or at least tolerate them. Group members often say that if they can "get it all out" in the group, they are not so distracted by these thoughts and feelings the rest of the week. The biggest mistake a therapist can make is to assist the group member in "covering up" such feelings by minimizing the emotion, too quickly asking the member about positive feelings they might have, or discussing an intellectual aspect of the situation. Instead, whenever the member begins to rush toward such distractions (often even apologizing for crying or having sad feelings), it is valuable to ask a few more questions about the feeling. "A moment ago you were starting to tear up. What were you feeling at that moment?" or "Telling us about that seems to make you very sad (e.g., angry/upset/frustrated). It must be difficult for you to deal with this situation." Inquiring further about negative feelings allows the member to more fully (a) air negative feelings that have been a source of conflict and a drain on them and (b) better tolerate these feelings, accepting that it is alright to have such feelings and that it is safe to express them in the group.

It is important for the therapist not to push too hard when eliciting a group member's expression of feelings. Simply offer an opportunity to explore. Point to the door, even open it a crack, but do not drag the members through. Overzealousness on the part of the therapist may result in a member having a rush of feelings that she is unable to integrate adequately, thus causing her to become more distressed than relieved, or the group member (and possibly other group members as well) might feel that she is being unduly pressured by the therapists or by the group. Ultimately, it is up to the group member whether and to what extent to explore frightening emotions. Another, more emotionally expressive person in the group can serve as a good model for exploring negative emotions. Often, members are concerned that if they allow themselves to express emotion (e.g., by crying) that "the flood gates will open and never close again." This fear will subside when they observe that other group members are not undone by expressing their emotions and can express their own emotions in more gradual and controlled ways. Members come to experience that the expression of feelings is usually a positive release, which leaves them feeling better rather than worse.

The group as a whole usually tends to become "informational" when difficult issues and emotions arise or following an especially emotional session. It is important for therapists to appreciate the emotional threshold of each person and the group as a whole. It may be important for individual members and for the group to be able to step back briefly from time to time. For the therapists, not "pushing too hard" includes allowing some lightness, humor, or more casual conversation to emerge before returning to more difficult topics. Yet returning to more difficult topics is important. The less therapists avoid difficult emotions, the less effort patients spend in avoiding them (see Exhibit 5.4).

Therapists also need to be aware of the dynamic range of affect regulation present in cancer patients. Many patients suppress feelings, afraid that once they begin to "let go" the "floodgates will open and never again close." Leading patients to express their feelings can be of value to them. Yet others are overwhelmed by their feelings, crying every day without relief. In this case, therapists can help patients get some

---

EXHIBIT 5.4

Leading to Elicit Underlying Affect

In response to Sarah's discussion of loss of sexual intimacy, Tahisha is explaining with little affect how her body has changed so rapidly in the last 6 months:

Tahisha: What with my mastectomy, hair falling out, going through the menopause all of a sudden, having no libido, and feeling irritated down there anyway, I don't really feel like a woman anymore.

Therapist: All that sudden loss of your femininity must be a real shock.

[If no response, then continue with]

It must make you sad to realize how much you've changed in just 1 year.

[Or to the group, if Tahisha cannot explore her negative feelings about it]

Has this sudden change in your bodies bothered you emotionally? How does it make you feel?

"cognitive distance" from the affect (see Exhibit 5.5). These patients can benefit from cognitive techniques, labeling their emotions, putting specific problems in perspective, and focusing on the moment at hand. Modeling derived from observing other group members will help them to naturally develop these skills.

Finally, a cautionary note: The therapeutic effort here should be to help patients uncover and tolerate strong conflicting feelings they have been afraid to bring to the surface. However, never assume such feelings exist and impose them onto patients. Every person's situation is unique, and so too is their ability to tolerate strong emotions. We must respect their unique situation in life and respect the power of the group to assist in the development of affect expression.

The three types of interventions mentioned above lead group members to express their concerns authentically rather than defensively. No matter what topics they are concerned about, expressing their concerns in a personal, specific, and affective manner ensures that the expression benefits the speaker and the group as a whole. We recommend that therapists lead group members to express themselves in the order presented above. In other words, it is helpful for members to personalize before being specific and to be specific before expressing affect. Otherwise a person could spend time being angry at the world for some ubiquitous injustice ("Why can't the government spend more on women's health!"). And even though their concerns may have some justification, little can be done about it in the group.

After a group member begins to express herself authentically, therapists can begin to ask questions that lead members to interact more fully with each other and to explore ways of coping better with the cancer and living more fully despite the cancer.

Fostering Active Coping

When group members discuss problems in a way that implies helplessness and lack of control, it is helpful to ask a question that leads them to explore ways that they can cope actively rather than merely give up in despair (see Exhibit 5.6). In reality, cancer patients do not have control over many things in their lives. Yet there is generally some way in which a cancer patient can be an active participant in coping with the problem. She may learn to react in a better way to the crisis, improve communication with others involved in the situation, and seek new ways to improve the situation itself. In general, when a member states that there is nothing she can do regarding her cancer, or some aspect of it, therapists can ask questions that lead the member to explore areas over which she does in fact have some degree of control. For instance, if a member states, "The doctor says that I have to go back for more

EXHIBIT 5.5

Leading to Distance Overwhelming Affect

If Tahisha makes the same statement as above but with eyes full of tears and saying she's cried about this every day for the past 6 months, therapists can respond with a statement that helps her focus on and gain cognitive control over overwhelming affect:

Therapist: Do you feel yourself focusing on the negative thoughts and feelings all the time? How would your life be if you were to focus on what you can do and can be?

---

radiation treatment. But it hurts so much that I just don't think I can take it again," the therapist might ask, "Have you tried discussing this with your radiologist or the technicians?" The therapist can also ask the group members (truly a panel of experts) for suggestions.

Rather than offering ready-made solutions to group members, it is almost always better to have group members find ways to actively seek

EXHIBIT 5.6

Leading to Active Coping

Wendy has been distressed about her feeling so fatigued and how this affects her work performance. Yet she has been mostly passive and expressing helplessness with regard to being able to do anything about it:

Wendy: Since I started this new chemotherapy I can't do the work I'm supposed to at the office. I'm tired all the time, can't concentrate, and look horrible. I can't afford to quit. If I keep taking sick time, I'll run out of sick days, and they'll start docking my pay. And anyway, the work just piles up for me to do when I get back!

Therapist: Have you spoken with your boss about your concerns?

Or, During these difficult times, what have you been doing to take care of yourself as best you can?

Or, When you've been sick before, or went on vacation, what did the office do without you?

Or, Sometimes we feel like we're trapped in a bad situation. We've been considering the problem from our usual way of looking at things. But these are unusual times, and maybe a different way of looking at things is needed. Let's ask others in the group if they've had a similar problem and what they did.

solutions and discuss them in the group. After all, if the goal is for members to develop active coping skills, then simply giving them advice makes for a poor learning experience. It is usually useful to follow a stepwise progression in leading members to explore active solutions to their problems. There is both therapeutic content to discuss as well as the process of intervention.

Therapeutic Process

- Ask questions that prompt the members to actively find a solution to their problems (e.g., "What can you do to improve the situation?").
- If this proves too difficult, it can be helpful to ask questions that bring principles of active coping to light (e.g., "How would you rather react to this difficult situation, in a way that would leave you feeling better afterward?").
- If this still does not lead to active exploration on the part of the member, the therapist can ask for suggestions from the group as a whole.
- As a last resort, it may be useful to gently challenge a group member, offering a nonthreatening interpretation of what appears to be a belief forming in the member and then asking the member or the group to comment on this interpretation. ("Sometimes people become more distressed when they feel out of control. I wonder if you are experiencing so much distress because you feel out of control with the treatment?" Or, "We all tend to see things from our own, somewhat limited perspective, especially in times of crisis when we fall back on what worked before. And it is difficult to consider other perspectives. But if our own way of dealing with a situation is not working optimally, it is useful to hear about alternatives that seem to work well for others. Has anyone in the group struggled with a situation like this, and found ways that seem to work for you?").

Group members are able to "normalize" their distress when they hear that others report feeling overwhelmed by events (i.e., they are experiencing a natural reaction to an abnormal event). Yet more often than not some group members can discuss ways they successfully cope with similar difficulties.

Change in times of crisis is always difficult, and therapists should not expect immediate insight and action. Over the course of the group, however, participants typically shift to a more active coping strategy, both cognitively and behaviorally. Of course, there are always individuals who seem to seek help and then reject the assistance they receive from the group. These and other difficult members are considered in chapter 8.

Therapeutic Content

In general, therapists can help group members to become more active in coping with their problem by asking questions that help them to do the following:

- identify the stressor and consider ways to improve the situation by altering the stressor if at all possible;
- identify their stress response, reacting in a way that would help them feel better;
- consider alternative solutions from their past, other situations, or from the group; and
- identify restrictive beliefs and consider alternative views. Gently challenge the patients' tendency to hold fast to their passive or restricted coping strategy, stating that in the midst of a crisis it is easy to lack perspective and fall back on habitual and limited ways of viewing and handling a crisis; ask the group for suggestions from their experience in similar situations.

Avoid Rescuing Patients

Whereas finding new ways of coping actively is an important focus of the group, it is equally important that therapists resist the temptation to move too quickly to solutions. Similarly, it is extremely important that therapists not allow the group to respond to expressions of distress by rushing to "fix" the problem. As mentioned earlier, it is often very difficult for group members (and for therapists) to tolerate the expression of other group members' painful and difficult feelings. Jumping in to fix the problem can be a defense against fully appreciating the painful feeling and experience associated with that feeling. The more fearful one remains of one's negative thoughts and feelings, the more one continues to be haunted by them day and night, and the more neurotic is one's flight to avoid them by grasping at any apparent solution that may come along. It is important that the therapists focus on authentic expression of thoughts and feelings and the capacity of each member and the group to take in, contain, and empathize with these internal experiences before moving to coping solutions. Except for severe acute traumas, being able to fully experience and express one's distress allows one to more fully move beyond it and to more fully explore all one's options.

Appreciating Individual Coping Styles

Therapists should appreciate that there are many ways of coping that may be healthy for different people to use. Some people need to feel as if they are in control over a situation before they can relax and live in the moment. Others feel a need to relax and live in the moment before they feel "clear-minded" enough to contemplate what they should do. Both approaches are valued and are fostered in the group by beginning and ending each group meeting with a mind-clearing meditation, along with discussion of various ways to approach problems in the main body of the meetings. However, therapists need to be on the look out for members who are *hypervigilant* (i.e., rarely let go of their worries) or *hypovigilant* (i.e., rarely consider their worries). Discussing these extremes helps members to balance their active problem solving with the ability to temporarily suspend their problems and focus in the moment.

Adjusting to a New Lifestyle

One reason people suffer in response to life events such as breast cancer is that it is difficult to let go of previous images of themselves and their beliefs about their world and instead to reconsider themselves and their activities in light of their new situation (Spira, 2000). With the diagnosis of a life-threatening illness, disfiguring surgery, ongoing treatment that damages body tissue, decreased energy, and decreased functioning, a woman must make a tremendous readjustment, not only in her schedule and her activities, but also in her view of her rapidly changing self and her new life circumstances. It may appear that a group member who maintains her usual work schedule and as a consequence finds herself increasingly exhausted and frustrated should simply cut back her hours at work. Similarly, one may simply try to reassure a woman who is distressed about not being able to play tennis as well after her mastectomy that she will find other activities that she enjoys.

However, feelings of grief and loss regarding their former selves and former lives may underlie the difficulty many women experience in making these transitions. This is especially difficult for relatively young women, for whom menopause may have been induced by oncological treatment and hormone therapy and who may find themselves less interested in or deriving less pleasure from sex. For women whose attractiveness and sexuality has been an important aspect of their self-image, a mastectomy, loss of hair, dry mucus membranes, and loss of libido can be devastating. Many younger women find they can no longer function as mothers (to the extent they used to). Work performance and reliability suffer for many months, if not years, in the case of recurrent cancer. Identities as "wife," "mother," and "worker," all built up over decades and fundamental to one's image, are threatened. Letting go of such fundamental building blocks of one's self-image is never easy.

Most women do find eventually that even a terribly negative event such as breast cancer brings with it significant opportunities for change and new life-affirming perspectives. In general, however, these benefits seem only to accrue after patients experience a good deal of pain and grief about what has been lost. After all, only when we face a life-altering crisis are we forced to reevaluate our basic assumptions.

Although it is important to encourage group members to embrace the possible opportunities for reprioritizing their lives and living life in the moment to the fullest extent possible, they also should be reminded that there are probably no shortcuts to this goal. One of the functions of the group is to help women face and express their feelings about what has happened to them and what they have lost so that they can adapt and move on (see Exhibit 5.7). It is important that therapists guard against a defensive use of "letting go" (as in depressive hopelessness or narcissistic wound—"I don't care; It doesn't bother me; I'm fine") or a kind of convenient "spirituality" that arises to simply cover up the losses ("My faith will serve my needs."). Whereas some adjustment and new commitments are authentic (i.e., the results of accepting one's situation and consciously committing to a new lifestyle), others are the result of a defensive cover-up. Such defenses are shallow and can lead to renewed crisis in short order, requiring that the patient deal with both the false commitment and the breast cancer. Instead, an honest review of what has been lost (perhaps temporarily in the case of a first occurrence of breast cancer and often more permanently in the case of recurrent breast cancer) as well as what remains will provide a foundation for what can lead to a substantial sense of meaning, purpose, and value in these women's lives. After these women are able to fully accept and reflect on their losses and their new circumstances, their commitment to whatever attitude, spirituality, or activity they choose will be far more profound, meaningful, and long-lasting.

Indeed, existential philosophers from Nietzsche to Heidegger have claimed that it was only in the face of such crisis, when one's habitual assumptions are virtually ripped away, that one can finally move toward authentically committing oneself to activities that allow one to live most fully: A 12th century Japanese woman wrote, "Each Fall rain brings ever deepening colors to the leaves" (Yuasa, 1966). Perhaps this is why so many of us enjoy working with cancer patients. They are poised to cut through the mundane and can tackle the essence of life. Therapists can use several therapeutic interventions to facilitate this growth and adjustment to current circumstances.

Reflecting on Change

When the group addresses changes they are experiencing in their lives, therapists can ask simple yet profoundly stimulating questions such as

- What has been lost (in yourself; in your lives)?
- What remains of value?

EXHIBIT 5.7

Leading to Facilitate Adjusting to Life Circumstances

Maria was a 46-year-old married dance teacher whose children had grown and moved away. She had mentioned that she had felt an "empty-nest" depression when her second daughter moved out last year before the cancer was diagnosed, but throwing herself into her teaching helped to give her a new focus and energy. Maria had a type of breast cancer that has a poor prognosis, spreading rapidly and requiring continued radiation and chemotherapy.

> Maria: Well, I'm not feeling so good. The treatment is making me really tired, and I've got bad sores in my mouth. But until this week it hasn't stopped me from teaching several classes a day. Then, yesterday, I find out that a student from my class went to the owner of the studio and begged her to have me stop teaching and find a substitute. So I've not been very happy today. . . .

> Therapist: That must be so disappointing for you. I know how much you've gotten from teaching dance, and if that's gone, then you must feel devastated [simple rapport]. First your children leave home, so you're not the same kind of mother anymore, and now you're not the same kind of dance teacher anymore . . . [focusing on the loss to facilitate the grieving].

[Then, after offering sufficient rapport and acknowledging the grief] Who are you if you are not teaching dance?

Or, What remains of value in your life when the teaching is not there anymore?

Or, What will you do to bring that degree of purpose and meaning to your life?

* * *

Vicki was a 48-year-old software engineer who was happily married to a successful businessman, had no children, and was diagnosed with a recurrence of breast cancer 4 months ago. She had been complaining how exhausted she was and how work was becoming increasingly difficult for her. When the group suggested she quit work, her responses ranged from how much they depended on her to her sense of "giving in" to the cancer if she quit work. After a time, the group suggested trying to cut back to half-time for a while (just to get her strength back), and she agreed this might be a good, albeit temporary, solution. Vicki discovered that she really enjoyed her newfound free time. She was more rested, found plenty to do, and even went out and bought a small puppy.

> Vicki: I have some news to report. Last week I submitted my notice to the company, and I'm really looking forward to focusing on *my* quality of life rather than what my boss needs. Going half-time showed me that they really could get along without me (quite a blow to my ego), and that more importantly, I could get along without the job! They're giving me a good bye party next week.

> Therapist: Wow. That's quite a step. You've really accomplished a lot in the past couple of months. What recommendations might you have for others in the group facing a similar situation?

> Vicki: Well, I don't know what to recommend for others. But I can tell you that I was afraid to quit because I thought work was my life, and without work I would be "giving up." But I found I had a whole life "out there" just waiting for me. So I learned I didn't have to "fight the cancer" by working myself to death. I found out that the best way to fight the cancer is to not be afraid to live as well as I can.

> Therapist: What do others think about what Vicki just said about "fighting the cancer by living as fully as she can?" What ways do you fight to stay living as fully as possible?

▪ What can you do now and in the future that would bring you the greatest sense of meaning, purpose, and value?

Exploring Unconscious Beliefs

When a group member makes absolute statements about herself or the world that may have been appropriate for her life prior to the cancer (e.g., I am a mother and that means taking care of my family) yet interfere with dealing with the current situation that she is facing (e.g., sacrificing self-care in order to care for her family), it is useful to ask questions that lead her to consider alternative ways of perceiving a situation and acting within it (e.g., "Are their times when your husband or teenager can help out?"). Principles of cognitive therapy apply here. Whenever a group member makes a statement using absolute terms (*all, none, always, never*) or guilt-oriented statements (*should, must*), it is useful to consider whether this attitude limits her ability to fully function in her current circumstances. Statements such as, "I should not cry. Crying is always a sign of weakness"; "I should not think about dying. Thinking negative thoughts will make me die faster (or thinking only positive thoughts will help me live longer)"; and "Patients should not argue with their doctors (or patients cannot trust their doctors)" all reveal beliefs about life that may interfere with a group member's well-being. Other such self-limiting beliefs include

▪ "I have to do everything for myself."
▪ "I have to rely completely on my doctors to make me well."
▪ "I should act 'strong' and not cry. Crying only shows that I'm giving in to the cancer."
▪ "One should not show emotion around others."
▪ "Once I begin to open up, I will never be able to stop the feelings. They'll be too much!"
▪ "I have to do everything perfectly or it is not worth doing at all."
▪ "I am what I do. If I stop working so hard, I will be less of a person."

Such beliefs about life are rarely considered consciously. They are usually developed in childhood and built up over a lifetime. It is not the purpose of this type of therapy to delve into childhood dynamics in any depth, nor to attempt to alter basic personality structure. However, when a woman's assumptions about self and life interfere with her ability to live more fully in her new situation, momentarily reflecting on these assumptions can help her to become aware of how she may limit herself and help her to consider alternative responses. Asking if others have noticed similar kinds of beliefs about themselves or the world can make for lively and therapeutic discussions.

Letting go of old self-images or assumptions about life to adjust to the current situation is certainly difficult. Yet the extent to which group members can reconsider their self-image and assumptions about life determines their ability to find what is of greatest value and meaning to them in the current situation.

Three methods of intervention can be useful for helping women to do this in the group:

1. *Challenge the belief.* The therapist can directly challenge fixed beliefs that interfere with current quality of life. This can be done by (gently) probing for other ways the group member can perceive a situation or act within it. A member may say, "I am a teacher. And I am not going to let the cancer defeat me, so I am not going to let anything interfere with my teaching schedule." Yet if it is clear that she is becoming increasingly distressed over her inability to teach full-time while receiving medical treatment, the therapist might ask, "Being a teacher is obviously important to you. What else are you, besides a teacher? What else brings meaning and purpose and value to your life?" If the group member is able to engage in such a discussion, such statements can be followed up by asking more difficult questions, such as, "If you could not teach any more, what would you do that would allow you to live as fully as possible?" Addressing such existential questions allows the member to put her life into perspective and to reconsider what is truly of greatest value to her in her life.

2. *Ask the group for alternatives.* Modeling (Bandura, Blanchard, & Ritter, 1969) is a powerful aspect of group therapy. Asking the group for alternative ways of viewing a situation or acting within it is a powerful way of showing a woman with fixed beliefs that her view is just one among many. This is especially valuable because most people are not aware of the assumptions they have about themselves and their lives. By opening a discussion in the group about ways that other group members view and respond to a particular situation, the member is helped to see her previously unconscious assumptions and can begin to consider the situation from an entirely different perspective. For instance, in the example given above, therapists could ask the group, "If you could no longer work in your profession, how would that affect you, and what can you do that would allow you to live as fully as possible?" Or, "What changes have you gone through since the cancer has arisen: What have you lost and what have you gained?"

3. *Use structured exercises.* To encourage individual members or the group as a whole to further explore existential issues implicit in

the concerns they raise, it can be useful to ask a series of probing questions about these specific issues. Some therapists prefer to use paper and pencil questions, which the members can reflect on for a few minutes before writing down their thoughts. Other therapists prefer to ask the same questions through dialogue, going to the next question when the group has sufficiently considered the prior question. The latter is more natural, but the former can ensure that every member participates and has an opportunity to adequately address each issue.

The use of structured exercises should be conducted with caution, however, because when therapists take charge of the session structure and topics, they shift the focus away from the group members. If exercises are used frequently, the tendency to rely on such structure is increased. However, when the discussion turns to self-image or assumptions about one's life, for example, and the group appears to be having difficulty reflecting creatively about these issues, a series of existentially oriented questions may stimulate deeper discussion. Thus, used sparingly, and when the issues are naturally emerging from the group, structured questions can be just what the group needs to allow them to reflect on intimate concerns.

Such questions might arise when group members make two types of statements:

1. *Statements that address the changing self.* Therapists should ask questions that help members appreciate that the self is fundamentally changing over time, in response to circumstances, and this is healthy and adaptive:
   - "You seem to be talking about changes in the way you see yourself." (This may include positive or negative aspects of body image, personality characteristics, beliefs, things you do, people you know.)
   - "How accurate is this self-image? For example, what was your self-image like when you were 20 years old, and how has that changed?"
   - "How much of your self-image was developed by circumstances, and how much has been a conscious choice?"
   - "What do you hope your self-image to be 6 months from now, or 10 years from now?"
   - "Over your lifetime, have some aspects of your self-image been 'true' and others 'false'?"
   - "How does your self-image affect what you do and how you do it?"
2. *Statements that make absolutist assumptions about self, world, or others.* When therapists suspect that a member's fundamental beliefs are

limiting their ability to live as fully as possible, given their new circumstances, they might ask the following questions:

- "I wonder whether that belief (characteristic, attitude) might be negatively affecting your quality of life."
- "When was this belief formed, and did this belief serve you well at that time?"
- "Does this belief still serve you well now?"
- "How does this belief limit you now?"
- "What alternative belief, attitude, or characteristic would complement the old habit belief and help you grow beyond the limitations of the old belief?"

These and other probing questions may be of use in challenging fixed assumptions that make it difficult to adjust to current circumstances. Several other existentially oriented structured questions and exercises (such as helping one to appreciate what one has lost and what one still has; reprioritizing commitments) are included in the Appendix.

Encouraging Supportive Relationships

One of the benefits of group therapy is that it offers members the opportunity to express emotions about their condition, as well as a chance to give and receive support within a community of people whose experiences are somewhat similar to their own. Therefore, therapists should make every effort to have this expression be directed toward another group member or to the group as a whole (see Exhibit 5.8). Two aspects of leading to supportive relationships are considered here: (a) interaction within the group and (b) interaction with others in one's daily life.

Facilitating Interactions Within the Group

Therapists should be wary of turning a group into a series of individual expressions or conversations with the therapist. Typically, the therapist should be relatively silent in this type of group. When needed to get a member or the group "back on track," they typically ask between one and three questions before yielding to another person or opening the discussion to the group as a whole to maintain an interactive discussion among members.

In general, when a member is expressing, but not relating, the therapist may use several methods to elicit interaction. The therapist can facilitate interaction with the following participants:

- *The therapist:* It may be helpful for the therapist to establish a connection with a group member by asking questions (eliciting per-

---

EXHIBIT 5.8

Leading to Encourage Supportive Relationships

Bethany: I like coming here because I can tell you all my worries that I can't share with anyone else.

Therapist: It's great that you can share your worries here. But I wonder, do you share these thoughts and feelings with your husband also?

Bethany: Well, of course I share a lot with him, but not everything. He's got enough to worry about without my making him worry more by taking on my worries, too.

Therapist: It's nice that you are looking out for his well-being. But I wonder if that's maybe keeping you a little bit apart at a time when closeness and support is so valuable?

Bethany: Well, I just don't want him to worry. His worrying won't make my cancer go away.

Therapist: Let me ask you, if your husband was feeling sad for some reason, would you want him to hide it from you?

Bethany: No, not at all. I've always been there for him. I'd want to help in any way I could.

Therapist: So why are you robbing him of that same opportunity to give you support and to be there for you?

[And later]

How many of you here find it easier to give support than to receive support?

---

sonal, specific, and affective statements about her distress and ability to cope with it). Following a member's statement that is external, abstract, or intellectual or a statement that shows evidence of passive coping, the therapist should probe for more authentic types of expressions in two or three questions and then redirect the next question to the group or to another group member to commence a dialogue among group members.

▪ *The group:* Therapists should normally limit their interaction with an individual group member to just a few questions and responses before asking the group as a whole to get involved. It is useful for the therapist to briefly summarize what the member has said (e.g., "It sounds as if you have been finding it difficult to get your concerns across to your doctor"), followed by statements such as, "Has anyone else had a similar difficulty?" or perhaps, "Does anyone who has faced these same difficulties have some advice for (member)?" This is useful not only when the therapist has been active for a time, but also when one or two members have been dominating the discussion. Making a summary rapport statement and then branching out to the group shows respect for those who have been speaking but at the same time models the importance of bringing everyone into the discussion.

▮ *Another member:* Whenever possible, it is beneficial to facilitate an interaction between two group members. This direct member interaction is an ideal way to give and receive support, and it helps to establish more direct and intimate relationships among group members than can be established between an individual group member and the therapist or between a member and the group in general. Therefore, following a group member's statement, the therapist can attempt to establish a two-way conversation for a time, before redirecting to the group: For example, "Sarah, you told us last week that you were finding ways to tell your doctor your concerns about reconstructive surgery. Can you offer any suggestions to Jodie that might help her out in her current situation?" After some discussion, "Jodie, do you think the way Sarah handled her situation could assist you in your situation?" This approach is especially effective if therapists can have two group members taking roles that help themselves and help each other. Consider a group in which one member is very quiet and tends to ask for help and then rejects it, whereas another member is very free in giving advice to others yet rarely discusses her own situation with the group. It would be very useful if the therapist could facilitate a discussion where the "quiet" member is able to use her experience to offer advice to the "helper" member, who would be encouraged to reflect on this advice.

Therapists typically find it easier to facilitate interaction in the order presented above (initially with the therapist, then to the group, and finally with another member). However, these are presented in reverse order of value to the group members. Interactions with other members of the group are in many ways superior to interactions with the therapist. This is evident from the common experience of group leaders, who often find that although they may give advice, it is only when another group member offers similar advice that the member receiving the advice becomes excited and decides to act on the suggestion.

Facilitating Relationships Outside the Group

Many interpersonally based therapy groups steer away from discussing relationships outside the group (Yalom, 1985). In group therapy for breast cancer patients, however, patients' relationships in their daily lives should be a focus. Issues of communicating needs to family, friends, coworkers, and medical staff as well as prioritizing time and commitment to different relationships are sure to arise frequently in group discussions. Hearing about the various ways group members interact with others in their lives helps all group members expand their options. Too often we get into habits of relating to others that are suboptimal. Focusing on a wide range of relationship issues serves to

1. Convey that different types of relationships require different rules (e.g., how much to disclose about one's cancer).
2. Clarify whether members are relating optimally in each situation (e.g., if the member is able to get what she needs or says she needs).
3. Teach skills to improve communication with others in one's life (e.g., "Sally, can you pretend that I'm your doctor/coworker/husband? Now, what do you want to say to me?").

In one of our groups, the discussion turned to sex, and several women in the group had a similar story to tell. As Jamie put it,

> When I came back from the hospital following my mastectomy, my husband was a little unsure about how to approach me. I guess I saw his hesitation and took it personally. After all, I wasn't the same woman any more. That, and I was sore there, so I didn't really feel intimate just then. So I suppose he saw *my* hesitation and pulled further back, and I saw *his* further hesitation, etc. So we just never got around to being physically intimate again. We never talked about it. We still love each other and snuggle, but the sex isn't there anymore.

After this discussion, several group members reported the following week that they had broached the topic with their spouses for the first time since the cancer was diagnosed.

Often such dialogues bring up associated issues of beliefs about giving versus receiving support and fear of seeming vulnerable. These are all good material for further discussions about how we relate to others. Once again, the therapists can rely on the expertise in the group for examples of how to improve one's interpersonal relationships.

Discussing spouses and family issues when there are single people present should not be avoided. Asking those left out of the discussion how such discussions affect them may uncover feelings of loneliness, regret, loss, or the need to form new supportive relationships. As in every other aspect of therapy, asking questions that reveal what is truly present under the surface should not be avoided.

FACILITATING FLOW

It cannot be emphasized enough that when the group is interacting well and members are expressing themselves authentically, no therapist intervention is required. However, when intervention is required to assist a member's exploration of issues or to get the group back on track, it is generally best to ask particular group members two or three questions before redirecting to the group as a whole. The order of questioning depends on what is lacking in the group member's statement. In general, it is probably a good idea to ask a group member first to personalize her subject, and then to specify the object of discussion, and finally to inquire about affect (depending on what is lacking in their expression). Once a person is expressing a concern in personal, specific, and affective terms, it is then useful to explore active coping and ways to better adjust to the new situation. However, the therapist should only attempt one type of lead before redirecting to the group (see Figure 5.1).

Therapists who wish to pursue a line of questioning with one particular member (rather than posing a question to the group in general) should wonder whether the line of questioning (a) is relevant to the group as a whole (and this individual work might serve as a positive model for the group) or (b) is likely to lead to a real breakthrough for the member, which would be well worth the group's time to wait for a few minutes while the member does her personal work. Even when the answer is yes to either of these questions, individual exploration should be limited to a few minutes. Group interaction is in many ways preferable to continued dialogue between one member and the therapist.

Because much of the power of the group lies in group interaction, a general guideline to follow is that each therapist should have about a dozen questions that she or he can ask during the entire group encounter. Therefore, each question must be selected with care and timing. Clearly this will not be the case in the first several sessions, where the therapist might need to ask up to 20 questions to model the flow of the sessions. Still, toward the final sessions of the group, the therapist might actually ask far fewer than 12 questions (about one question every 7 minutes or so), because the group will be doing most of the good work on its own. This is as it should be, because an important goal of therapy is for group members to learn how to explore their own situations outside of therapy in ways that are initially introduced and explored in the therapeutic encounter.

General Guidelines

In addition to the specific methods of facilitation described above, some general guidelines are helpful to keep in mind. It is useful to have an existential and experiential focus in the group, and to remain a facilitator of the process rather than a lecturer or individual therapist (see Table 3.1).

THE GROUP CULTURE

Typically, within 4 to 6 weeks, the group as an entity begins to emerge. It may be noticed as mutual support. It may be seen in the group setting itself against the leader (a "we" [patients] and "you" [therapists] mentality). Or it may simply be noticed as an intangible feeling of caring in the entire group. Often it is noticed by its later absence for a brief period of time. This feeling of the group as an entity unto itself will help each member feel that she is part of something greater than herself. Members will begin commenting on how important the group is to them, and they will reschedule appointments or even vacations so that they will not miss the group. Such a culture arises naturally. Therapists can interfere with the development of this culture, however, if they are too active in the groups. The group that centers on the therapists has much more difficulty forming the type of supportive culture that so benefits each member. Thus, although therapists are initially central to the group (in forming cohesion and modeling the style of exploration), they must rapidly recede into the background, emerging only when necessary to get the group's process back on track.

EXISTENTIAL FOCUS

The therapeutic process we described allows for authentic examination of existential concerns, without having members feel that they are participating in the psychological "games" that may characterize some approaches. Because issues are driven by group members, discussion stays close to the concerns of the members. Process facilitation by the therapist assures continued authenticity in members' quality of expression. In addition, this process can facilitate members' ability to be more fully "in the moment" rather than linger in the past or worry about the future. In general, there are two major existential emphases to this therapeutic approach:

1. *Facilitating authentic expression and action.* Rather than assisting to cover up painful thoughts and feelings by supporting habit beliefs and actions, or too quickly focusing on the "positive," therapists facilitate
   - recognizing and challenging limiting habitual self-image;
   - tolerating honest feelings and thoughts, including grief and loss of prior self;
   - examining what personal qualities or activities would bring the greatest meaning, purpose, and value to one's life; and
   - commiting to these activities or personal development.
2. *Being in the moment.* Therapists can encourage patients to spend more time focusing on each moment rather than spending ex-

cessive time and energy on the past or worrying about what terrible things might occur in the future. For example, therapists might ask what percentage of one's attention is in the moment as opposed to the past or future. Therapists can point out the following:

- We enhance what we attend to. If we pay attention to our worries, then we tend to worry more. If we attend to what we are doing in the moment, then we are more fully present in that moment.
- Our bodies and minds support what we attend to. If we attend to our worries, our body and mind become aroused to support that perceived emergency. If we attend to a comfortable sensation, or what we are doing, then our body and mind become calmer and more focused.
- It is worth focusing on our worries if we can act to improve them. If there is nothing we can do, continuing to focus on these worries simply perpetuates them. When there is nothing we can do to correct a situation, it is better to focus on what we are doing in the moment or on some comfortable sensation.

Example exercises for these ideas can be found later in this chapter and in the Appendix.

GIVING ADVICE

When facilitating discussions, therapists must avoid the trap of answering questions definitively. Instead, they can draw on the knowledge of the group, which is a superb source of expertise. In educational groups, therapists are teachers relaying information. In group discussion, however, the therapists' emphasis should be on facilitating the process, not providing content. *The Breast Cancer Notebook: The Healing Power of Reflection* (Stanton & Reed, 2002) contains a great deal of information and provides references to many additional information sources. If managed well, providing information in this way should assist the therapists in staying out of the "expert" role. When the therapist does become the expert, it is often extremely difficult to return to facilitating the process —the group simply does not permit the therapist to shift gears. Avoiding giving advice may be difficult for a therapist with particular expertise, but it is also critical to stay clear of this role. The expert–therapist should find ways to diffuse questions, such as suggesting that the group member speak with her oncologist or that the subject could be discussed after the group among individual patients. This approach focuses members' attention on the group process rather than the group becoming an informational meeting (and correspondingly diminished in terms of interaction among members in personal, specific, and affective ways).

EXPERIENTIAL EMPHASIS

Part of what distinguishes this approach from typical psychodynamically oriented and long-term psychotherapy groups is the attitude toward therapeutic interpretation. In this approach, therapists steer away from abstract psychological interpretations about members' statements or group process. Similarly, therapists avoid overtly analyzing the personalities of an individual. Instead, therapists comment on

- structural aspects of the group (e.g., "We have about 15 minutes remaining. Is there anything anyone wants to say that you didn't get an opportunity to?" Or, "We've been meeting now for 8 weeks, and I'd like to take this opportunity for us to reflect on how the group's been going for you. What has been beneficial so far, and what would you like to get from the group in the future?"). Such meta-group comments allow the group to reflect on where they are and where they wish to be. In fact, this may serve as an experiential metaphor for similar reflections about their lives. It further gives group members a sense of ownership and control over group process. This type of reflection also assures them that the therapists are monitoring the contextual group structure so that they can focus more fully on their individual needs.
- topics overtly manifesting in the group (e.g., "I notice that there has been a lot of discussion about lack of control this past hour. Losing control over one's health must be very frustrating, and a little scary"). Summarizing group themes can help members focus more clearly on the issue at hand. Following a summary with a concrete question can then turn the focus back on the members to continue doing their "work." ("In what ways have you lost control, and in what ways have you found some measure of control in these areas?")
- process occurring in the group (e.g., "I notice that everyone has been attempting to help Janice with her problem. How does that make you feel, Janice?"). Commenting on the group interactions can help to reveal what is happening as well as provide a pause for reflection. In this case, Janice might have felt embarrassed, harassed, or pressured to change at a time she may not have been ready to. She might have felt support and caring from the group she might not have previously felt. Therapeutic comments on such group process interactions can offer a momentary pause that allows examination of whether the process is healing or hurting.

Caution must be used with this type of structural, topic, or process reflection, however; the therapists must not be seen as a "head shrinker," someone sitting in the corner analyzing everything that is said. Although such reflections as these are occasionally useful, it is far more useful to offer the members an opportunity for direct experience, allowing them the opportunity to "live their experience" rather than to have it merely commented on.

Therefore, therapists should look for situations where the group members can experience a problem and solution firsthand in the group rather than merely commenting about it. Rather than attempting to point out habitual ways of thinking and then asking a member to reflect about the beliefs that may underlie this way of thinking, therapists can offer an opportunity for the member to directly experience healthy ways of dealing with a problem (Mitchell & Everly, 1993).

If Alice is having difficulty with her husband understanding some of her needs, the therapist attempting to foster reflection and awareness of personality patterns might say, "I notice (or you've said) that you sometimes have difficulty expressing your needs and problems here in the group, as well. Is this a common pattern in your life? In what other situations does this pattern arise?" This line of questioning might be useful in a cognitive–behavioral psychotherapy group that attempts to make unconscious patterns conscious. In groups facilitating emotional expression and support among cancer patients, however, it might be more useful to say, "Sometimes it's hard to let others know what you need. Is there a way you can let those of us in the group know what you need, so that we can better understand what you're going through?" Or, "Julie, do you know what Alice needs? Alice, can you let Julie know what your needs are?" Thus, rather than stimulating reflection about one's patterns, therapists should look for an opportunity to encourage a group member to experience directly her restrictive way of coping and try out a healthy alternative in the group. A reflective remark after such an experience has far greater impact than a remark stated in the absence of such an immediate experience. Moreover, when the experience is strong enough, such reflective remarks are often totally unnecessary.

THE ROLE OF HUMOR

Humor that arises naturally in the group can be an important addition to therapy. Humor is an important part of our life experience and, as a reflection of group members' lives, the group should reflect this aspect as well. Allowing humor to arise can help group members feel closer to one another, help put problems in perspective, and offer a break from an extended period of bleakness. Yet therapists should exercise caution when introducing humor. The therapeutic role is an important one, and if overused, the attempt by a therapist or group member to "lighten the atmosphere" can send a message that consideration of difficult material is only tolerated so long and only to a certain limited level of affect.

(Indeed, members often even apologize for crying or complaining!) Therefore, humor naturally arising from the group should be applauded, but only when appropriate. When clearly distracting from some serious work on the part of members (either others or the person making the joke), the therapist can demonstrate appreciation of the humor through a rapport statement but then remind the member or group of what work they were doing. "It's good to be able to have humor about the topic. But I'd like to get back to what Marilyn was saying about her discomfort in dating. Marilyn, when do you plan to disclose that you've had breast cancer and a mastectomy?" Thus, occasional jokes or laughter from a member, the group, or the therapist can be humanizing, but inappropriate use can be distracting and limiting.

FACILITATING ACTIVE COPING STRATEGIES IN LIGHT OF PERSONALITY STYLES

One unique feature of human beings is the extent of our adaptability. We are the only creatures who can live in every climate on earth, in isolation or in huge communities, in agrarian or combative environments. The ability to have a range of personality characteristics makes this adaptability possible. Indeed, Jean Piaget (1990) defined *intelligence* as the ability to adapt. However, the personality characteristics one develops to adapt in a particular environment are not necessarily adaptive in drastically changing conditions. Such is often the case with women diagnosed with breast cancer. It is valuable to assist group members in recognizing their coping styles built up over many years and to assist them with developing a greater repertory of skills that will help them in their current situations.

Rather than attempting to explore and displace restrictive personality patterns, this approach to therapy instead helps group members to add skills to their repertory with respect to their personality. Which skills are developed depends on the current needs and personality of each member. In many cases, specific strategies that have worked well for a member throughout her "healthy" life may not be optimal when she has to cope with life-threatening illness. Moreover, when faced with such a crisis, members tend to cling to ways of coping that worked previously. Therefore, above all else, it is important to respect members' current style of coping: It helped them survive to this point and still helps them to some extent. However, when a group member is having new difficulties functioning in some aspect of her life, especially when she is using a habitual way of responding that may contribute to the dysfunction, therapeutic support may be required. This therapeutic support comes in the form of asking questions of the member or the group that will help the member to consider alternative skills that may help to balance the skills she currently possesses. (See section Fostering Active Coping, earlier in this chapter). These alternative skills may offer additional resources that patients can draw on in these new and challenging circumstances. Such skills are especially useful when the member is perceived by the therapist or group as using one extreme dimension of coping.

The dimensions outlined in Table 5.1 serve as examples of how the coping strategies of group members can be viewed as falling along a continuum. Therapeutic emphases intended to assist group members in broadening their repertoire of resources are suggested for each dimension.

Topics Discussed in Breast Cancer Groups

Whereas therapists continually monitor the process (i.e., the quality of group members' expression), the members themselves naturally focus on specific topics of concern. Group members typically raise certain issues (related to their treatment, physical health, and psychophysical coping); therapists can ensure that other issues of concern are also raised at some point. The topics that group members address are based on their personal concerns, whereas the issues raised by therapists are based both on issues that patients in other groups have found relevant (e.g., sexuality) and on scientifically determined risk factors for worsening quality of life and physical health that group members may not otherwise bring up on their own (Table 5.1). Given sufficient time, group members typically raise most issues, but therapists should use every opportunity to ensure that all of the following topics receive adequate attention.

Topics most commonly discussed in groups include those of concern to the group members and those deemed of value by the therapists. Topics generated by the members stem directly from members' immediate needs and concerns, such as coping with pain, nausea, sleeplessness, negative mood, intrusive thoughts, and physical fatigue; improving appearance; and improving communication with doctors, family, and friends (Speice et al., 2000; Spiegel & Spira, 1991; Spira, 1991). Addressing these issues early and often helps to establish rapport with group members. As Maslow (1968) argued so convincingly, one must take care of basic functional concerns before one is able to adequately address existential issues.

Member concerns are often concrete topics of interest that can be discussed directly and easily in a group. Issues of greatest scientific concern, on the other hand, focus on process-oriented skills that may re-

TABLE 5.1

Therapeutic Strategies for Improved Coping

Coping style	Problematic (excessively passive)	Optimal (balanced)	Problematic (excessively active)
Emotional:	Flooded with feelings: no control over time, place, or extent of expression. Therapy: The structure of the group supports members' internal structure; offer opportunities to have member feel group support; distance the overwhelming problems (e.g., cognitive reflection can be further distanced by having the group explore issues the member raises; affective exploration can be postponed).	Open affect: willing and able to express positive and negative feelings with some measure of control over time, place, and extent of expression. Therapy: Reinforce how useful this strategy has proven to be for the member.	Repressed feelings: overcontrolled and rarely expressing. Therapy: Probe affect; use others for modeling affect expression; set tone of "normalcy" of affect expression in and out of group.
Cognitive:	Overwhelmed: unable to put issues aside. Therapy: Establish the ability to focus calmly on what is occurring in the moment (where there are few things that are distressing); emphasize group support.	Open: willing and able to consider any issue on occasion. Therapy: Reinforce how useful this strategy has proven to be for the member.	Avoidant: unwilling or unable to examine issues. Therapy: Calmly focus on issues; use group to model exploration of difficult issues.

Focus:	On the past: regretting what one did or missed doing. Therapy: Address feelings about the past and ask what one can learn from that experience to improve one's current activities.	On the moment at hand: Spends most of one's conscious attention focusing on where one is and what one is doing now and in the near future. Therapy: Reinforce how useful this strategy has proven to be for the member.	On the future: worrying about what might occur. Therapy: Focus on what one can act on to improve the situation, and let go of what one cannot act on at that moment.
Self-efficacy (control):	Helpless: no confidence in control of one's destiny. Therapy: Focus on what one *can* control.	Moderately confident: can control some aspects of one's life, and coping with cancer. Therapy: Reinforce how useful this strategy has proven to be for the member.	Overconfident: and overcontrolled in one's efforts to determine one's destiny. Therapy: Inquire about real issues that lie out of one's control.
Hope:	Hopeless: lack of or distorted hope for future. Therapy: Focus on what one can find of value right now.	Hopeful: flexible optimism, hoping for the best but being able to prepare for and adjust to worse outcomes. Therapy: Reinforce how useful this strategy has proven to be for the member.	Restricted hope: only will believe and consider positive outcomes. Therapy: Ask what would happen if not everything goes according to plan in the future.
Social support:	Isolated: no functional or emotional support. Therapy: Get member actively participating in this group and other groups.	Adequate: sufficient functional and emotional support, wisely chosen from among ample resources. Therapy: Reinforce how useful this strategy has proven to be for the member.	Overwhelmed: burdened by too much network contacts and the inability to say no to unwanted favors. Therapy: Learn to say no.

Table continues

TABLE 5.1

(Continued)

Coping style	Problematic (excessively passive)	Optimal (balanced)	Problematic (excessively active)
Vigilance:	Uncontrollably Dissociative: spacing out or overfocused on irrelevant detail in the face of distress. Therapy: Controlled dissociation with distanced reflection of coping with distress (as in self-hypnosis).	Controlled awareness: focusing on immediate environment and critical issues, yet being able to reflect and recuperate, as necessary. Therapy: Reinforce how useful this strategy has proven to be for the member.	Uncontrollably hypervigilant: obsessively attentive to problems, worries, or sensations. Therapy: Controlled dissociation with distanced reflection of coping with distress (as in self-hypnosis).
Humor:	Humorless: no perspective; overly obsessive. Therapy: Encourage some lightness from time to time; get member involved when this occurs in group.	Appropriate humor: perspective on situation with occasional lightness. Therapy: Reinforce how useful this strategy has proven to be for the member.	Comedic: inappropriate or constant lightness. Therapy: Probe serious issues.

quire professional facilitation. Topics emphasized by the therapists are often emotionally difficult for members to pursue at the time, even though they may well feel better after the group meeting. These include issues of establishing meaningful social support, confronting fears, expressing negative emotions, and seeking control over what can be improved while letting go of what cannot be controlled. Although members may avoid discussing or expressing negative emotions or issues, they generally benefit and appreciate when this does occur. In our experience, discussing these difficult issues in the group helps members to focus on living more fully in each moment, without as much distraction during the rest of the week. Moreover, directly addressing the difficult issues of illness and dying assists group members in re-examining the way they live, which gives them the opportunity to choose to spend more time in activities that are more meaningful and valuable to them.

Rather than focusing on what is discussed, the therapeutic style leads members to examine these aspects of their lives. Therapists must gently lead group members into exploring difficult realms, lest they meet resistance and lose the trust of the group. The best leader is usually one who can follow the group, gently introducing new ideas within the context of members' relevant experience (Roter et al., 1995). Exactly what, how, and when topics are discussed varies greatly depending on the special issues raised by group members. The use of *The Breast Cancer Notebook*, as well as the process facilitation described earlier, should help balance the scientific concerns with the concerns of the group members.

The following is a brief overview of topics commonly discussed in breast cancer groups of the sort advocated here. This list of topics and issues discussed within those topics is derived from an analysis of 16 meetings of a mixed first occurrence and recurrent breast cancer groups, using a grounded theory approach to qualitative analysis of triumph, (Glaser & Strauss, 1967) and confirmed by interrater reliability (>.75) among four independent raters (Spiegel & Spira, 1991; Spira, 1991). Topics are presented here in terms of frequency of discussion (as generated by group members), which can also be seen as being listed from the most social to the most personal.

SMALL TALK

When the women enter the therapy room, they most often engage in small talk. This might be about the parking situation, or how crowded the freeway is getting and tricks for avoiding the worst traffic, or perhaps a good movie they have seen recently. It is not unusual for several small group or dyad conversations to start up. Someone who mentioned she would be experiencing an important event might be asked about it.

These are normal and healthy exchanges, until the door closes and the group begins. When the group begins, small talk should be minimized. It is common for the group to drift back into small talk. However, therapists should redirect to whatever topic was being previously discussed or to a new topic of importance as soon as possible.

INFORMATION GATHERING AND SHARING

There is often some housekeeping to discuss at the beginning of a group (usually after the opening meditation). Therapists or group members will want to acknowledge or inquire about absent members or to mention who will be unable to attend the next meeting. There is often some general medical information that members wish to share or other announcements of common interest. ("Next week there will be an American Cancer Society Walkathon, and I'm signing people up. Any takers?")

It is good to get this information sharing out of the way at the beginning of the group and then to say something along the lines of, "O.K. Let's begin. I mentioned last week that we would continue to discuss with Mary the difficulties she is having at work. Mary, ..." When information sharing of this sort erupts in the middle of the session, it is best for the therapists to acknowledge the topic and then to redirect to an issue of therapeutic value. Occasionally, when the group or an individual member begins discussing a general and impersonal informational topic with enthusiasm (e.g., a new cancer treatment in the newspaper that day), it may be necessary to let it continue for a minute or two and then to suggest that they can continue to discuss that topic after the session ends, because group members can do little about that in the session, followed by "I wanted to get back to what Jenny was saying about . . ."

MEDICAL STATUS AND TREATMENT

Personal issues regarding medical matters often arise, and they are well worth discussing. Economic problems (e.g., insurance, copayments, the need to continue working) are topics that arise frequently. Patients are typically concerned with the fundamentals of living (shelter, food, and money) before they are able to focus on other quality-of-life issues. Satisfaction with their medical treatment is also a topic that is likely to be frequently raised. Members are likely to compare notes on the procedures they have had and the doctors who treat them. Sharing of cancer information of a personal nature is also of value, because it is most often on their minds. Patients undergoing treatment will want to discuss side effects, hopes for improvement, and any new treatments they are undergoing.

These treatment and medical status issues are well worth discussing in the group. In fact, there is no way to avoid them; these issues are uppermost in the minds of patients undergoing treatment. The conversations are valuable as long as they focus on a member's personal and specific situation, with therapists tapping into their reaction to and ways of coping with it. However, therapists must continually be vigilant lest the discussion become external, abstract, and intellectual. Discussions about medical status and treatment can offer a bridge into exploration of coping and adjustment and be an opportunity to draw other "experts" into the conversation, facilitating group bonding.

DOCTOR–PATIENT RELATIONSHIP

Also quite commonly and easily discussed is the important relationship between a woman and her medical team. Therapists can assist in helping patients to clarify the role they expect the physician to play in their lives. Some patients see clearly that the physician is merely one person doing what he or she can to assist them in their treatment, whereas others raise the physician to near deity status and cannot understand why the doctor does not simply make the cancer go away. Also commonly heard are statements about how one likes or dislikes aspects of a physician's approach. Some members focus on reputation for competency, whereas others express preference for a doctor who is compassionate and a good listener. Communication difficulties with one's treatment team arise quite frequently; a common concern among patients is miscommunication with physicians and lack of sufficient communication among the treatment team.

Therapists can assist group members by encouraging active and open communication with members of the medical team. Occasionally, role-playing in the group can be a helpful practice. Hearing how others have improved their communication with their doctors can also help motivate those experiencing difficulty. As with facilitation of all topics, appreciating the diversity of what each group member expects from their medical support should be emphasized, with care taken to avoid one person foisting her expectations onto others in the group.

FAMILY AND SOCIAL NETWORK

Communication and relationship issues also commonly focus on one's family. Family relations can become stressed over economic matters, changes in physical intimacy, fears of what the future holds, what to share with family members, and many other issues. Often, the patient is reluctant to share her intimate feelings and thoughts with her family members out of a fear of distressing them further.

Therapists should consider helping group members to become closer to their family through advocating open honest communication whenever possible. In some families this does not work at all. Most often, however, openness and honesty help both the patient and the family to become closer and grow more loving during this difficult time. One therapeutic device that is exceedingly simple yet rarely considered by group members is to ask what the family member wants to know.

Relationships with friends, coworkers, and community groups (e.g., church, PTA) can be more complicated. The group member may want to share some information about her illness or recovery with some friends or coworkers but not with others in her life. The social stigma associated with having cancer has lessened over the years, but patients must decide individually how much to share and with whom. Sometimes "reverse stigma" occurs, with many wanting to offer advice to the cancer patient. After all, sharing information is a socially acceptable way to deal with a crisis, but "just being there" for a friend or acquaintance's emotional needs is much more difficult to achieve.

The group discussion can help tease out those with whom sharing would be valuable and the type and extent of sharing to allow. Therapists can also raise issues of re-examining relationships, with more emphasis going toward those relationships and groups that result in greater personal meaning and distancing oneself from those that are less important or overly fatiguing.

GROUP THERAPY ISSUES

Less commonly raised by group members and less easy to discuss are issues related to the group process. Matters including group cohesion, asking for and offering support, and evaluating the group process are occasionally brought up by patients, sometimes as criticisms, other times as positive comments about what they value in the group. Occasionally, a group member may want something else from the group (e.g., more positive thinking or information about cancer) and express frustration with the emphasis on personal expression. At other times, a group member may make a statement (often in the context of another topic under discussion) about the value of the group for her.

Therapists should encourage all such expressions of the impact of the group on members' lives. In fact, therapists should periodically initiate discussion on how the group is going. This encourages the members to reflect on where they want to go in the group and in their lives. It also gives members a sense of ownership and direction over the group.

ILLNESS-RELATED COPING SKILLS

Although cancer patients are often quick to point out their problems in coping with their illness or treatment, it is less common for them, at least at the beginning of therapy, to also discuss ways of actively coping with these problems. Asking about ways to actively cope with the problems raised is often the purview of the therapists. Aspects of illness-related distress include psychological and physical stress, hopelessness, negative feelings, loss of control, pain, insomnia, and fatigue.

Therapists can help by listening and showing appreciation of the difficulties faced by cancer patients, and then gradually steering the discussion toward what one can and cannot control. The meditation exercises can help with sleep and reducing pain and overall psychophysical stress. In addition, encouragement from therapists and other group members for ways of handling illness-related difficulties can be a strong incentive for developing hope and active coping strategies.

ISSUES RELATED TO ILLNESS AND DYING

Patients with a first occurrence of cancer fear a recurrence of cancer, which most often means dying within a couple of years. There can also be a mix of emotions about having cancer, including guilt about being ill or even guilt about feeling fortunate when another group member has a downturn or dies. Patients with recurrent cancer have all of these feelings, but in addition they have to consider practical arrangements regarding their deaths, such as financial, legal, hospice, and funeral arrangements.

One of the most important roles therapists can serve is to allow the time to grieve for one's own and others' bad news about their cancer. If a member dies, it is especially important to allot time to discuss what that person meant to each person in the group, possibly pointing out what she has given to and received from any member who wishes to speak. A fitting goodbye may take the form of an imagery or hypnosis exercise, in which each woman imagines something of value the member gave her and then to imagine something that she gave the deceased. In general, discussion about the death of a member, or of death in general, can reduce the stigma and fear.

Occasionally, the discussion turns to suicide. A patient may express something along the lines of, "When the time comes that I can no longer be self-sufficient, and I'm a burden to others and in terrible pain, I will choose to end my life." Such discussion should be facilitated openly and calmly by therapists. However, therapists might want to point out that most patients who say this early on rarely if ever follow through with it. This is because pain can almost always be controlled with medicine and exercises, and most patients are self-sufficient right up to the last week or two of their lives. Furthermore, it is rare that family members do not feel gratified by helping someone who has helped them so much in their lives.

SELF-IMAGE

A common and inherently intimate topic raised by group members is that of changes in the way they define themselves. For many, this begins with changes in body image caused by cancer treatment, as well as how one looks and feels. It can also include the way one defines oneself in terms of what one does (e.g., functional roles, activity level, ability to fulfill one's commitments). Cancer affects practically everyone's self-esteem; for those who already have issues around their worth and value to others, this experience can greatly magnify their worries. Having cancer can greatly influence one's aspirations—we often define ourselves in terms of what we plan to do, and now these plans must be put on hold. In some cases, past negative experiences of illness (of one's own illness or that of a loved one) can come rushing back, influencing one's current feelings about one's own cancer.

Therapists should take every opportunity to flush these feelings out. Many of them can be detrimental ("My aunt died of breast cancer when I was 12, and I really don't want to end up like her, all pale and wasting away"), whereas others can be quite positive ("All my life I've defined myself in terms of my work. Well now I realize that I'm *not* just my work"). These issues occasionally rise to the surface, but other times they lie just beneath the surface, waiting to emerge. When patients make statements that point to changes in their self-image, it is useful to ask overtly about what this means for them ("You said that you don't feel very valuable anymore. Valuable to whom? How do you define your value?"). Such discussions can lead to improved self-worth, a self-definition that goes beyond the surface, and consideration of deeper life values.

LIFE VALUES

Although it is often stated that the diagnosis of cancer can be an opportunity for growth, this opportunity is frankly usually only undertaken by those who have completed their primary treatment. For those still in treatment, merely coping with daily events takes most of their mental and physical energy. Yet those who can begin to "settle down" a bit from the crisis of diagnosis and treatment often naturally turn toward deeper issues in an attempt to put their lives in perspective. The exception to this "rule" is patients with recurrent breast cancer, who might be receiving constant treatment and who do not know if they will survive the next year or two. Faced with possible death, it is natural for such persons to turn toward larger issues as well. Although group members may be somewhat reluctant to bring up such topics or to pursue them in much depth on their own (topics rarely raised in casual conversation), they invariably appreciate the opportunity to explore these issues.

Issues that go beyond daily functioning and coping and which strike at the heart of who one is include religious, spiritual, and philosophical beliefs about what one is when one's self-image, activities, and daily commitments are being stripped away and what it means to die. Reflecting on these issues can help to gain new perspective on where one should place one's values and energy. It can lead to enjoying life more fully in each moment, reflecting on one's life, altering one's views of or recommitting to what is important, and in many cases improving one's sense of being in the world.

Therapists should make every effort to facilitate such discussions by keeping the conversations on such topics after they have been raised by group members. Therapists can also ask questions to steer members toward such conversations whenever possible: "Sally, you were talking about how much you have changed since the cancer was diagnosed and how you're a completely different person. Can you tell us what remains of you and your life now that so much has changed, and what will remain even as you get older or possibly sicker?" Group members remember these kinds of discussions long after the group ends and feel as if the group has had lasting value, beyond simple coping with daily activities.

OTHER TOPICS

There are a variety of other valuable topics that can be discussed in the group. Those mentioned above are most commonly heard, but therapists should not shy away from other topics of importance to group members and of value to exploring their personal, specific, and affective relationship to it.

However, as is continually emphasized in this approach, the quality of expression is more important than what is discussed. Therapists should be less concerned with the topic than ensuring that patients are expressing themselves authentically (personal, specific, affective), exploring active ways to cope, adjusting to their new circumstances, and interacting productively with others in the group and their lives.

Experiential Exercises: Relaxation, Meditation, Self-Hypnosis, and Imagery

A third element of the group meetings is the teaching and practicing of experiential skills. These skills, when practiced both in the group and on one's own, help members to

- feel more personally comfortable (allowing them to explore difficult issues with assurance that they will be able to return to a baseline comfort);
- feel more comfortable in the group (facilitating bonding with others as the therapist leads them through these self-comforting exercises, which can allow them to feel they are getting some immediate and concrete benefits rather than awaiting the more nebulous benefits that come over time from group discussions);
- increase their benefit from therapeutic discussions (as they can reinforce the topics through the experiential practices); and
- increase their ability to cope with worries and psychophysical symptoms, as well as their general sense of control over their cancer and their lives (because they can do something whenever they like to reduce their negative feelings and thoughts and improve their general sense of well-being).

As described, each group therapy session begins and ends with a relaxation exercise. Besides training group members to develop these skills, beginning and ending each group session with a relaxation exercise helps to increase members' confidence that no matter what arises in the groups, one can always return to this calm, comforting state. These exercises also constitute ritual transitions into and out of the psychological focus of the group.

In general, it is useful to begin with an exercise that is more meditative in nature (breath awareness, sensory focus, self-comforting) and end with a longer relaxation or imagery exercise, where the imagery might relate to some topic that was just discussed in the group (e.g., control, self-image, communication, saying goodbye). Therapists should feel free to use a variety of techniques with which they may be familiar and which they feel may be helpful for group members. However, unless at least one of the cotherapists has training in hypnosis, it is better to begin and end with a simple breathing relaxation that can be refined over time. Exercises should always emphasize group members' ability to manage their own experience during the relaxation exercise, and the exercises should not be overly directive in nature. It is helpful to emphasize the group members' ability to find this quiet state of relaxation on their own when they wish to. We never use techniques that suggest some specific control over the disease process (e.g., imagining one's immune cells attacking the cancer), because such approaches can install false hope and have never been proven to be effective. Instead, we use methods that have been proven to improve quality of life. Some examples of specific techniques follow. Others are included in the Appendix.

RELAXATION WITH MEDITATION

A 5-minute relaxation coupled with Zen meditation can be helpful in settling down and beginning to concentrate on important issues (see Exhibit 5.9). In fact, the inability to dismiss certain concerns from one's mind can serve as the basis of discussion for that session.

These exercises are referred to as the *Opening* and *Closing Relaxation*, a label chosen to be as accessible and nonthreatening as possible. During the first group meeting, the therapists should inform group members that a variety of relaxation techniques will be used at the beginning and end of each session. Multiple techniques are used because people typically find that certain types of exercises work better for them than others. If a particular technique is not effective for a group member, it is likely that she will find others over the course of the group that are better suited to her. Therapists should explain that the effectiveness of relaxation techniques improves with practice, and they should encourage participants to practice them at home, as well as describe a variety of situations in which these techniques might be helpful (e.g., having difficulty falling asleep, feeling overwhelmed at work, when receiving chemotherapy). If a participant does not wish to participate in a particular exercise for any reason or wishes to stop at any time, she is asked simply to sit quietly during the exercise.

Group members are encouraged to practice whatever technique works for them on a daily basis, but at no time is the use of relaxation exercises treated as a homework assignment, nor are participants asked to keep records. However, handouts can be given for review. Therapists should discuss the relaxation exercises periodically over the course of the group therapy, inquiring about participants' experience with them in the group and their use of these or similar techniques outside the group. The intent of these discussions is to find out about group members' experience, to answer questions, and to provide problem-solving assistance and support. That is, participants are invited to use the relaxation exercises to the extent they find or believe that they may improve their quality of life; they should never be told that they must do them

EXHIBIT 5.9

A Standard Relaxation/Meditation Technique

The following is a standard relaxation/meditation technique (Spira, 1994) that is simple to learn yet highly effective. It should be read slowly and softly.

Initial Relaxation

Squeeze your hands, raise your shoulders, squeeze your eyes shut, and take a deep breath in, as deep as you can ... and then release, let go of all your tension, your breath flows all the way out, and you can sink down into your chair.

Feel gravity helping your body to relax down into your chair:

- Feel the weight of your legs, letting gravity pull the weight of your bones toward the floor ... and then let the muscles relax, as if they are "melting down" along your bones ...
- Feel the weight of your pelvis, sinking into the chair ... your muscles melting and your pelvic organs sinking down into the chair ...
- Feel the weight of your abdomen settling into your pelvis and all your abdominal organs relaxing and letting go ...
- Feel the weight of your spine resting into the pelvis and all the muscles of your back melting like warm honey ...
- Feel gravity allowing your shoulders, lungs, and heart to sink down toward your abdomen ...
- Let your eyebrows relax and sink toward the floor, let your jaw release, and allow all the muscles of your face to melt a little bit ...
- Allow your head and even your brain to relax down toward your shoulders. . . .

Meditative Component to Clear and Focus the Mind

As your body continues to relax and rest and feel comfortable, focus on your breath.

- Notice the air flowing into and out of your nose ... notice the change in temperature as the air flows in compared to when the air flows out ... notice the change in texture as the air flows in compared to when the air flows out ... notice the place that the air touches in your nose and throat as the air flows in and out ...
- If your thoughts or feelings distract you, notice that distraction, let it go, and come back to feeling the breath flowing into and out of your nose.

Feel this calm soothing flow of air for about 10 breaths.

- Place your hands on your chest ... notice how your hands rock forward as your chest expands with each inhale and returns back to your center with each exhale ... notice how your elbows are gently expanded out to the sides and then released back toward the center ... and you may even be able to notice how your back gently expands into the chair behind you and slightly releases the pressure on that chair with each breath ...
- There's no need to make any effort to breathe. Rather allow the breath to happen effortlessly, as if the breath is breathing you. In fact, to help you release your excess effort to breathe, at the bottom of each exhale let the breath out just a little bit more, relaxing it out as much as possible, before the inhale begins anew.

EXHIBIT 5.9

(Continued)

Feel this gentle massage from the inside, as if a balloon is expanding and releasing effortlessly, for about 10 breaths.

- Place your hands over your lower abdomen . . . feel the warmth of your hands merging with the warmth of your belly . . . allow that warmth to float forward and backward, effortlessly, soothing and comforting . . . allow that warmth to spread, soothing and comforting your whole body . . .
- Imagine the breath to be centered in your pelvis, expanding down and out (like a balloon effortlessly filling and expanding in all directions equally), and then easily releasing, letting go of any tension, any effort, any pain. Each inhale is as fresh as the first breath you've ever taken, and every exhale is as precious as the last breath you'll ever take.

Feel this soothing rocking of the warmth, back and forth, for about 10 breaths.

Finally, simply sit, feeling your body expanding and releasing effortlessly, silently, soothingly. If your attention is drawn away by a thought or a feeling or a sound, simply notice that your attention is being pulled away, let go of that distraction, and absorb yourself as fully as possible in the body expanding with every inhale and releasing with every exhale.

The meditation exercises usually end in the following way:

- It's nice to know that you can return to this state of relaxation and calm focus any time you need to or want to, simply by doing this exercise. And you can bring this comfortable feeling back with you now, as you . . . (with voice increasing in volume, pitch, and speed) feel your chest raising during the inhale . . . and with the next inhale or the one after, you can . . . (with voice increasing in volume, pitch, and speed) raise your eyes and eyelids up toward the ceiling, and then focus back in the group feeling clear and calm and alert.

This simple breath meditation takes only about 5 or 6 minutes. It is useful to practice when first waking up. When you drive to work, you can sit in your car for 5 minutes and do this breathing exercise before you go on to face the day. It's useful to practice this for 5 minutes before lunch. And when you drive home it's helpful to sit in the car for 5 minutes and do this exercise before you go on to begin your evening routine. Finally, it's valuable to do this exercise just before going to bed.

Note. An ellipsis (. . .) indicates a pause of about 3 seconds.

or that the exercises influence the course of their disease. Participants who wish to have an audiotape to assist them in using these techniques are given information about commercially available tapes. We have discovered that some members increase their use of relaxation techniques dramatically, whereas others choose not to use them outside the group context. At a minimum, however, the relaxation periods provide a quiet space before transitioning into and out of the group.

SELF-HYPNOSIS

Self-hypnosis can be conducted to increase a sense of personal comfort, reducing physical or mental distress. From this comfortable base, one can consider issues that might otherwise be difficult to address. Any topic discussed in the group or done in one of the structured exercises could be material to be examined in this state. A typical format would be to induce a light trance and imagine an event in the distant future. One can imagine what it would be like to deal with it in the "old, problematic way" and then to imagine what it would be like to interact with it in a "new, optimal manner." Methods of self-hypnosis for the medically ill patient have been described in detail elsewhere (Spira & Spiegel, 1992). Training and experience are required to use any form of hypnosis effectively. After patients have received this training, self-hypnosis at the end of a group can help them address the issues raised in the group in a way that leaves them calm and feeling that they have addressed important issues at a deeply honest and open level (see Exhibit 5.10).

Hypnosis has three phases. The *induction phase* involves suspending one's vigilance (to current time, environment, causal logic, and self-awareness), resulting in becoming more fully absorbed in past memory or future fantasy. In the *utilization phase*, the individual accesses past or current resources relevant to some current problem and creatively applies these resources, addressing the problem in a new and successful way. In the *integration phase*, the individual imagines a more successful scenario in the near future and runs through the new scenario in her imagination.

Hypnosis differs from typical relaxation techniques, which merely focus on shifting from a state of sympathetic arousal to parasympathetic recuperation (although those undergoing a hypnotic induction report that it is very relaxing). Hypnosis also differs from Eastern meditative traditions, because meditation (e.g., Zen) involves attending to and becoming absorbed in sensation, such as light, sound, and feelings without effort to conceptualize and corresponds to alpha EEG rhythms. It also differs from visual imagery exercises, which commonly maintain a sense of reflective awareness and problem solving (beta EEG rhythms) while imagining more successful ways of addressing some area of concern.

Hypnosis is a normal and natural state, which we go in and out of several times during the day (e.g., daydreaming, drifting off to sleep, driving down the freeway and exiting at the correct exit without really thinking about it). It is helpful to address difficult areas that have been too difficult to fully acknowledge and to generate new creative ways to handle a particular problem.

EXHIBIT 5.10

Self-Hypnosis at the End of the Group

For example, if the discussion has centered on issues of control, the following self-hypnosis exercise may be appropriate as a summary of the session:

1. *Establish a comfortable base:* Induce a state of relaxation and comfortable absorption. (See the Appendix for an example of a rapid induction method.)
2. *Consider negative aspect:* "While you continue to let your body and mind relax, imagine a scene off in the distance, where you have no control over some aspect of the cancer. Notice what you are doing in that scene . . . how you look, how you sound, how you feel." [Pause for about 20 seconds]
3. *Return to baseline comfort:* "Now just let all the images and feelings from that scene go, and return to feeling comfortable and relaxed." [Pause for about 5 seconds]
4. *Consider positive aspect:* "While you let your body and mind relax, now imagine a different scene off in the distance, where you have some control over some aspect of the cancer, or coping with it . . . Notice what you are doing in that scene . . . how you look, how you sound, how you feel."
5. *Summary and future suggestion:* "It's nice to know that, like many aspects of life, there are aspects of your cancer over which you have little control, and others over which you do have some control. It's good to recognize the difference, and then to put most of your efforts into what you can control. So, next time you find yourself focusing exclusively on what you cannot control, remember to also consider what you can control."

Other examples of hypnosis exercises and techniques are included in the Appendix.

IMAGERY

Imagery exercises can also be conducted independently of trance induction, after inducing a state of simple relaxation (following, say, several minutes of progressive muscle relaxation or breath awareness). In this case, it is important to make the exercises very simple and not to rely exclusively on visual imagery. (Approximately 20% of people report an inability to create visual images.) Simply contrasting two situations may be sufficient. For instance, following a brief relaxation: "Imagine speaking with your doctor about some important subject, but in which the doctor isn't communicating in the way you'd like. What do you look like, how do you feel, what emotions arise in you." (Pause for 10 sec-

EXHIBIT 5.11

Summary of Therapeutic Facilitation

Specific Interventions

Therapists need not intervene when the group is interacting effectively. However, if the interaction drifts from optimal quality of expression, therapists can facilitate group interaction by

- asking questions that lead members to authentically express their concerns (in a personal, specific, and affectively integrated manner);
- asking questions that lead the members to explore alternative ways of actively coping with their problems, adjusting to present circumstances, and improving interpersonal relations in the group and in their lives; and
- teaching meditative and reflective techniques that group members can also use on a daily basis.

General Principles

Therapists maintain a therapeutic culture in the group through emphasizing

- existential themes, reinforcing discussions that have a bearing on what is of greatest meaning, purpose, and value in patients' lives;
- experiential opportunities rather than mere reflection about or psychological analysis of issues that arise;
- the expertise of the group rather than their own advice;
- a range of affect, including occasional humor as well as crying; and
- the development of coping skills that complement one's current tendencies.

Common Topics

Themes commonly discussed by groups and which therapists may wish to further facilitate include

- medical status and treatment
- doctor–patient relationship
- family and social network
- issues pertaining to the therapy group
- coping with one's illness
- death and dying-related issues
- self-image
- life values

Experiential Exercises

- meditation
- self-hypnosis
- imagery

onds.) "Now imagine a different situation where you ask things in a way that makes the doctor explain things in a way that works better for you. How do you look and feel in this situation? Compare and contrast these two situations in your mind." Similar contrasts can be suggested for poor versus effective communication, passive compliance versus active engagement, and so on. Virtually any topic can be reflected on in this way. It is important to end each imagery session with a minute of simple relaxation, emptying the mind of thoughts and attending to a comfortable feeling in one's body.

Thus, visual imagery is similar to the simple hypnosis exercise discussed above, but it uses a simple relaxation and does not focus on induction of a state of suspended vigilance and a high degree of absorption. Certainly, some people will go into a trance during imagery exercises, whereas others will have a clear awareness of themselves doing the imagery at this time and place and for a specific purpose. Fortunately, the imagery exercises can be beneficial for both types of people. Simple relaxation plus contrasting two ways of operating in a situation is effective in helping the group members to integrate what occurred during the group. Making the imagery exercise too complex detracts from its value and makes it difficult for group members to learn to practice this on their own. Moreover, it is detrimental to lead the group in a specific series of images (e.g., go to the beach, see yourself on a mountain top) because some members will inevitably have a negative reaction to this image (e.g., burns easily, fear of heights). Rather, it may be useful to ask group members to imagine themselves in a situation that is most comforting for them, and leave it at that (see the section "Moderate Trance Induction" in the Appendix).

Summary

This chapter has offered general principles and specific therapeutic and experiential interventions to facilitate optimal group interactions. It also reviewed themes commonly discussed in the groups (see Exhibit 5.11).

Conclusion

This chapter has provided the "meat" of the therapeutic style suggested in this book. The following chapters include ways to strengthen the intervention through supportive tools, addressing problems that can arise in the group, and extensions of this approach to other populations.

Typical Problems in Group Facilitation

6

The therapeutic methods described in the previous chapters are effective for facilitating the majority of groups and patients. However, problems are bound to arise. Therefore, we now turn to facilitating difficult issues that typically arise in the group and difficult group members.

Problems Arising in Groups

What follows are some situations that commonly arise that therapists should be prepared to handle.

GROUP ISSUES

Down Time

It is important for therapists to be able to tolerate periods of "down time," or silence, in the group. It may be necessary for group members to struggle through some period of silence, awkwardness, and anxiety before taking consistent responsibility for initiating and managing their own discussion. However, it may occasionally be necessary for the therapists to stimulate discussion when the group appears to be floundering. If down time occurs too frequently, it almost certainly signals an over-reliance on the therapists to provide the group with material. On those occasions when it appears to be necessary for the therapists to stimulate discussion, one way to get things moving might be to ask, "If the group were done, and you were on your way home, is there anything you wished you might have said or done in the group that would have made you feel better, or would have made your time here more meaningful?" The therapist might wonder aloud about a group of women who have had breast cancer finding it difficult to think of anything to discuss. If all else fails, the therapists may introduce a specific exercise likely to stimulate conversation afterward. It can be helpful to ask about something they found interesting or disturbing in *The Breast Cancer Notebook: The Healing Power of Reflection* (Stanton & Reed, 2002) or else to introduce an existentially oriented exercise. (A few examples of existentially oriented exercises are provided in the Appendix.)

Multiple Topics

If several important issues have been raised by one or several group members, the therapist can ask a question concerning one of the points to get the group to explore this area more deeply. The other points can be addressed at a later time. Or the therapist can simply state that several points have been raised and that they are all important. The group can be asked to decide what topic to address first, giving members a sense of control over the group.

Late Surges

Group members frequently attempt to get everything in during the final few minutes of a meeting. Too much intensity at the end of a meeting can make it difficult for the group to end. This is especially the case if the intense experience comes from an otherwise introverted member finally opening up to the group. Yet it is important to hold to the agreed-on group structure and to give the member and the group as a whole a chance to wind down and to integrate their feelings and thoughts. One way to handle this situation is to affirm the importance of the member's expression and to suggest that the group might begin with this topic at the next meeting. If the emotions are very strong in general at the end of the meeting, acknowledging this beneficial expression and then using a relaxation technique to help members settle down before leaving can help them experience firsthand that emotions can be expressed and then allowed to subside.

Illness, Recurrence, or Death

When a member becomes ill, has a recurrence or complication, or dies (a very rare occurrence in groups for women with primary, i.e., first occurrence, breast cancer but unfortunately all too common in recurrent breast cancer groups), the emotional tone of the group will obviously turn quite sober. In fact, this can have a mobilizing effect on the group. Such tragedy rapidly cuts through denial about the seriousness of one's illness and helps focus members' attention on issues they may have been avoiding, such as fears of losing control, death, losing one's family, unaccomplished goals, and so on. Learning to deal with a group member's tragedy is a model for coping with one's own losses and fears of death.

Subgroups

Cliques are bound to form within a group. This is to be expected, because some members will find a natural affinity with certain other members' views or styles. Such bonds can be very useful in establishing social and emotional support. Unlike psychotherapy groups, members of cancer groups are encouraged to see each other outside the group meetings if they so desire to foster supportive relationships. As long as extragroup activities (e.g., social events) are kept out in the open, there should be few problems. However, if one subgroup gangs up against another person or subgroup, then the therapists must step in. For example, intragroup hostility may occur when a subgroup of active problem solvers attempts to help another member "too much" or when there are honest philosophical differences between members (e.g., as in the role of "positive thinking," prayer, alternative medicine). In such situations, therapists can point out the benefit that different people obtain from different approaches, the value derived from having a wide range of options from among which each member may select, and the importance of respecting this wide range of options.

Being Single

Discussing spouses and family issues (including sexuality) when there are single people present should not be avoided. Asking those left out of the discussion how it affects them may uncover feelings of loneliness, regret, or loss, and the need to form new supportive relationships.

Conflicts Among Group Members

Conflicts among group members arise in several ways. Most often they occur when members disagree on ways to approach a problem. The therapists should step in and defuse the disagreement by pointing out that there is no single correct way to approach a problem. There are as many different approaches as there are people, and the group provides much-needed diversity. Members should be encouraged to listen carefully to the approaches of other members for future reference. Other interpersonal conflicts arise from frustration with individual personalities; these are discussed in the next section.

Conflicts With the Therapists

There are several ways in which group members can come into conflict with one another or with the therapists. This may occur if the therapists are perceived as having agendas that are contrary to those of the members of the group (see Exhibit 6.1). Conflicts can also occur if the therapists do not adequately brief the group about the style and goals of the group process (and review these goals from time to time), if the therapists are lax in their efforts to establish and maintain close rapport, or if the therapists are perceived as being in conflict with one or more members with whom other members of the group have an affinity.

EXHIBIT 6.1

Example of a Conflict Between a Patient and Therapist

Jodi was a 38-year-old single mother with recurrent breast cancer. She was very eager to discuss positive thinking and any alternative medicine approach for beating the cancer. She worked from 6 a.m. until midnight without a pause, driving herself literally to distraction, so that she did not have to confront any negative thoughts or feelings about her illness or the possibility (probability, given her prognosis) of dying.

The therapist prompted her to relax and discuss her fears, but she only wanted to discuss ways to overcome the cancer through positive imagery, flying to England or Mexico to try alternative treatments, and so on. The therapist tried to voice the purpose of the group as attempting to uncover both fears and hopes that may be influencing one's actions or lack of actions, but she was very clear about just wanting to focus on the positive and avoid the negative. Jodi eventually dropped out of the group. She died 5 months later.

The therapist could have been less directive with her, offering more reflective rapport on all her activities to help her see the extremes she was going through to avoid negative feelings and thoughts. Yet would she have stayed in the group and begun the process of living more comfortably and fully in the moment, spending more quality time with her daughter and making peace with herself? Or, would catering too much to her desires have altered the group for the other members, detracting from benefits they might have eventually derived from the group? Would voicing that there were several different ways of coping with having cancer have accommodated both? There is no clear answer to these questions. But knowing the range of responses helps to make more informed decisions in difficult situations like this.

These potential conflicts must be avoided. Adequate briefing should occur from the time of recruitment right through the course of therapy. Maintaining rapport should always be a primary function of the therapist, with reflective listening, summarizing, and nonverbal cues used liberally. Group members inevitably disagree with one another at one time or another, but they should be able to see that therapists handle these disagreements with respect toward the member in question and toward the group as a whole. (If a problem arises primarily with one individual and it cannot be simply and quickly resolved in the group, therapists may find it necessary to take the time to discuss the problem with the member outside of the group.)

Lack of Interest or Energy

Another source of problems in the group may arise from lack of stimulation rather than conflict. There may be times when the group simply does not offer anything to speak about or offers only material that would be appropriate chit-chat at a social occasion. In this case, the therapists must stimulate interest (see Exhibit 6.2).

On rare occasion, even these strategies do not stimulate discussion. In such cases, it may be better to completely "switch gears" and intro-

---

EXHIBIT 6.2

Therapeutic Interventions for Stimulating Group Discussion

In response to situations in which there is a seeming lack of interest in the group, the therapist can raise the following (from specific to general):

- Earlier we were discussing "X." I'm wondering if that is an issue for some of you who did not speak up. Jane?
- Last week, we began to discuss "X" but did not get a chance to finish the discussion. Have you thought any more about it? Jane, you were saying. . . .
- What are your reactions to the (psychoeducational) material you looked at this past week?
- You know, most groups are interested in discussing [e.g., sexuality, communication with physicians, fears of recurrence] at some point, but this group has not gotten around to it yet. How is [topic] going for you?
- Here is a group of women with a life-threatening illness and life-altering treatments. What might underlie the seeming lack of material to discuss?

Such questions should be followed by facilitating discussion in the usual way.

duce a structured exercise likely to stimulate discussion. Examples of structured exercises that groups of breast cancer patients have found useful are in the Appendix. These should only be used as a last resort, because dependence on such therapist-led and structured exercises tends to change the nature of the groups, with members relying more on the therapists for guidance, structure, and material. Still, as a last resort, they may fit well with the theme of the group and can serve as a strong stimulus to group members. Ample discussion should always follow such exercises, stimulated by asking a general question such as, "How was that exercise for you?" or in the very rare case that this also fails to stimulate interactive discussion, "What did you answer for Question 1?"

Controversial Topics

Topics frequently arise that are highly controversial, not only among medical doctors, but among group members as well. There are bound to be people who are very excited about something and want to proselytize its virtues, whereas others in the group, or the therapists themselves, are as vehement about its danger. Such topics include

- alternative medicine (either as an adjunct to or replacement for standard oncological therapy);
- new protocols (current research protocols, treatments that others may be getting, future "cures" for cancer, and so on);
- positive imagery for altering the immune system (e.g., imagining Ms. Pac Man eating up the cancer cells);
- positive thinking (avoiding sad and negative thoughts and feelings and instead thinking only good thoughts about getting well);
- God as oncologist (if one prays for health, God will grant health); and
- planning for suicide (when things get out of control and too painful).

In general, it is useful for therapists to express no overt opinion but to refocus on personal responses, motivation, and affective aspects of the issue: "What have you gotten out of praying for your health?" As always, it is helpful to comment on diversity, asking for others' opinions and experiences: "Have others here also prayed for their health? What do you believe this has given you?" It is sometimes useful to comment on such approaches as an effort to improve one's coping and hopefulness.

Some unique aspects of each of these topics warrant further comment.

Alternative Medicine

Alternative medicine represents a wide range of activities. These could include simple passive (e.g., massage, acupuncture) or active (e.g., Tai Chi Chuan, yoga, biofeedback) techniques to help patients tolerate treatment and improve general mood and quality of life. They can also include intensive diets, fasts, enemas, and substances intended to cure the cancer—sometimes to the exclusion of oncotherapy. In general, most physicians do not mind alternative or complementary methods that do no harm and that may improve quality of life for patients. However, when the treatment is so intensive as to be detrimental to the patient's quality of life (strong herbs, severe fasting, and coffee enemas that exhaust the patient) or when the alternative approach is intended to replace standard oncotherapy, the matter should be examined closely. Replacing standard medical or surgical therapies is extremely dangerous in the case of first-occurrence breast cancer, where the treatment can be highly effective and women are unlikely to survive without it. However, the effectiveness of oncotherapy in recurrent breast cancer is less clear, and patients may have a well-considered opinion about the continued use of chemotherapy or radiation for possible quality of life with no obvious survival benefit. In either case, however, it is imperative that group members be encouraged to consider all viewpoints and to keep their oncologist apprised of their actions. Such discussions in the group are helpful. A therapist's role is to help group members consider all options.

New Protocols

Group members often (and understandably) become excited when someone mentions a new treatment for breast cancer that is being tested or developed. Dealing with breast cancer is a struggle, and no one hopes more than cancer patients themselves for a cure. Although it is natural and expected for discussions to turn to this topic, staying there for any length of time or revisiting it frequently serves little purpose. It is important to acknowledge patients' hopes for a cure but then to turn the conversation to something they can discuss in personal and specific terms. One common method is to ask the group about how the topic of a cure one day brings with it the fear that they will not get this cure in time for their own disease. (This is especially relevant for women with recurrent breast cancer.) If they insist on continuing to discuss the new treatment, therapists can gently (and positively) encourage them to share this information with one another after the group and to attend instead to the immediate issues that members have raised.

Positive imagery for altering the immune system is common among cancer patients. Initially popularized by Carl and Stephanie Simington

(1995), positive imagery is a concept many cancer patients, feeling help-less in their treatment, find attractive because it gives them something to do actively to improve their health. Unfortunately, there is no evi-dence that such imagery helps the immune system fight the cancer or improve survival. There is evidence, however, that active coping is better than passive helplessness for the immune system (Fawzy et al., 1997) and reduces the incidence of breast cancer recurrence (Watson, Greer, Pryun, & Van Den Borne, 1990). Rather than denying negative emo-tions, a healthy acceptance of one's illness is correlated with improved quality of life and possibly increased survival (Taylor & Armor, 1996). Spiegel and Glafkides (1983) found that women with recurrent breast cancer improved their quality of life (and later argued for increased survival) despite addressing more negative than positive issues in their lives during the group therapy. So whereas specific imagery probably does not help improve the cancer, taking an active coping attitude along with honestly addressing important issues in one's life may help improve quality of life and possibly physical health. However, therapists must wonder (sometimes aloud) whether such imagery is an effort to deny the seriousness of one's illness, which is clearly not help-ful.

Positive Thinking

As with positive imagery, positive thinking, popularized by the work of Bernie Siegel (1973/4), has helped many women who have felt helpless and hopeless in the face of the disease to rally their coping skills to better confront their disease. However, positive thinking has been taken by many women to mean that they can overcome their cancer by avoiding sad and negative thoughts and feelings and instead thinking only good thoughts about getting well. This is not what Dr. Siegel intended (Siegel, Spira, & Ulmer, 1992; personal communication, December 4, 1993), and it is clearly not a healthy attitude for most women with breast cancer. Negative feelings and thoughts are an authentic and natural part of life and especially so when faced with a cancer diagnosis. To avoid such personal experiences is to avoid a major and important aspect of one's self and to feel increasingly inauthentic. Breast cancer treatment is al-ready an alienating experience. To further alienate oneself from oneself is a tragedy. Friends and family, also feeling helpless and wanting to help, encourage positive thinking. It is part of our culture to "fight" a disease by "bucking up" and not letting it get the upper hand. Whereas this attitude makes sense in dealing with major depression or in stopping the onset of hypotensive shock following a traumatic accident, it can be carried to extremes, to the point that feelings of sadness or fear can be discouraged. Therapists must reassure members that honest expression of feelings is a good and healthy thing. It helps them to feel integrated and authentic in their every action, to consider what is of greatest value to commit themselves to at this time, and to appreciate relationships more fully. Therapists who run cancer groups almost universally agree that the most integrated and authentic group of people they have ever met are women with breast cancer.

A cancer patient once said in the group that she

> was struggling with the concept of "fighting" the cancer. But what does it mean to fight the cancer? If I could see it I could try to beat it up. But it's elusive. So I fight it by being brave and not running away from it. Confronting it in myself, by allowing myself to cry when I am sad, ask for comfort when I am scared, and dance when I am happy. To me, that is fighting the best way I know how.

Another cancer patient described "positive thinking" in much the same way:

> Positive and negative thinking does not have anything to do with WHAT I am thinking about. It has to do with whether I push the thoughts and feelings away [negative thinking] or whether I am brave enough to allow whatever thoughts and feelings to arise and to consider them honestly [positive thinking].

God as Oncologist

Spirituality (the belief that one is part of a greater whole) is generally taken as being healthy for quality of life and physical health, and whatever path one follows to pursue one's spiritual beliefs should be encouraged. Patients usually do this instinctively, without encouragement from therapists. Yet occasionally groups include patients from a fundamentalist tradition who believe that if they pray for a cure for their cancer, God will grant them their wish. Furthermore, such people may tend to push this belief on other group members. This can be offensive; yet members may identify with being very religious and take offense at being told how to pray or what to pray about. In one group, in response to a question about what the women had been getting out of the group, one woman (Elizabeth) stated that she was not here to get anything out of the group but rather to let others know about God and how God could cure them if they asked him to. After an awkward silence, the group members were asked what they thought of what had been said. One group member replied, "I find it surprising that you [Elizabeth] presume to know what God had in mind for all of us. And, at any rate, I don't feel that I should ask for something from my selfish and limited perspective." Another member stated that she "takes offense because I consider myself to be a good Christian. Do you think that I don't pray correctly, and that is why my cancer is progressing? Or is it that I am bad and God does not listen to me?" Elizabeth was silent after these responses. However, group members also believed that people have a right to their beliefs, and an important part of the group is to learn from each other, so the importance of listening to everyone's views was emphasized. This helped defuse the tension, and the group returned to a discussion of the importance of spirituality in their lives and in coping with cancer.

Planning for Suicide

Therapists should expect that at least one member in every group will broach the subject of suicide at some point in their future. Primarily among women with recurrent breast cancer but also among women with a first occurrence of breast cancer, they talk about the possibility that they may commit suicide if and when the disease progresses to the point that

- they lose control over their bodily functions and mental faculties,
- they develop excruciating pain, and
- they become a burden to their families.

There are a great many "rational" reasons for and against suicide in the case of terminal illness. In the case of breast cancer (and most cancers), however, patients

- Do not become an excessive burden to their families. In our experience the families feel more of a burden when patients have died. It is the imagined burden that troubles the patient. Yet if her son or spouse was ill and he wanted to kill himself to spare her the burden of his illness, would she encourage him to kill himself? Quite the contrary—she would do anything to keep him with her.
- Do not become helpless and out of control, except for maybe the past few weeks or even days of their lives. No one can know when that time will come. Many women with recurrent disease go into remission for months or years, during which time they report extremely valuable relationships and experiences that they would not trade for anything.
- Do not become riddled with pain. In almost all cases, anesthetics and self-help techniques control most of the pain that comes with bone metastasis.

Our role as therapists is to make sure that this most important and potentially last decision of their lives is also the most fully considered. If they are depressed, or misinformed, then it is our duty to prevent them from acting rashly. That being said, however, there is little one can do to prevent a determined person from committing suicide. Yet in all the cancer patients we have seen in our groups and all the discussions about suicide, we have yet to see one group member actually take her own life. When patients get to the place they had feared, they realize that it is not nearly as bad as they thought it would be. They also come to even more intensely appreciate that each moment is precious and that they cannot simply throw it away.

FACILITATING DIFFICULT GROUP MEMBERS

Therapists can interact with the large majority of group members in the ways described above. However, one or more members in a group may require special management. In times of stress, we tend to fall back on old habits or personality traits that may have been useful once but are no longer optimal. Personality characteristics associated with interpersonal problems can be manifested in an especially strong way at this time in the group members' lives. Therefore, it should come as no surprise that some members are interpersonally disruptive in the group.

In general, it is best to attempt first to deal with a problem member within the context of the group, managing as well as possible to carry on, as long as she is not too disruptive. If this does not improve the situation, it may be advisable to discuss the situation with the member in private (before or after a meeting or on the phone). Of course, this should be put clearly and respectfully (e.g., "You obviously have a lot to share. Yet the point of the group is to let others express and find out what works for them, as well. I would like to find ways to allow all group members to have an opportunity to talk."). If this effort is unsuccessful, it may be necessary to suggest that the group may not be a good fit for the particular member (see the section on terminating a member's participation below). Pregroup interviews can help eliminate some but certainly not all of these problems. Even when pregroup interviews are not feasible, patients rarely have to be asked to leave a group; almost all issues can be addressed in the group setting.

Several types of difficult group members and suggestions for interacting with them are described below.

Excessively Introverted

Especially quiet, shy, or frightened members appear to prefer to receive benefit from the group by "osmosis." Yet these members may benefit more fully if they are drawn out in a safe way. Other, more expressive members can serve as models, followed by the therapist asking the introverted member if she has similar concerns. Therapists should seek any opportunity to have these members help others in the group. The added structure of the first three groups as well as the check-in and check-out procedures are especially helpful to facilitate interactions among quiet members. Yet additional attention to them is warranted throughout the group. Although not all members need to express themselves at the same level to receive benefit, therapists should be attuned to times when quiet members have something to share and give them the opportunity to do so.

Excessively Extroverted

Especially verbose, interrupting, or externally focused members must be managed lest they overtake and redirect the group in ways that may not be optimal. It is useful to allow some expression on the part of such a group member (she is a group member, after all). Yet when such members disrupt the participation of other members by monopolizing group time, it is important for the therapists to model an acceptable way of interrupting them politely and redirecting the discussion to the group or to another group member. One method is to say, "Excuse me, you've said a lot, and I just want to make sure I am following what you've been saying." Then the therapist can summarize in a sentence or two, get an affirmative acknowledgment from the speaker, and finally redirect to the group by asking whether anyone else has had the same type of experience. This serves to limit the speaker, make her aware that she should give others a chance to speak, and yet at the same time, affirms the value of what she has said. Occasionally, to limit the number of times certain members speak, it may also be useful to say, "We've heard a lot from a few people, but I'd like to give an opportunity to others to discuss their experiences with this situation."

As stated before, if such respectful yet pointed remarks are insufficient to curb a single patient's domination of the session, therapists should handle the situation by discussing the situation briefly with the patient at the end of the session. Also of concern is the reaction such members engender in the therapists. Some degree of irritation is natural, and even valuable, as it alerts the therapist to feelings that others in the group may be having. However, it would be wrong to let this irritation show. Keep in mind that practically every group will inevitably have one or two people who tend toward verbal excitation or need to control the group. Expecting and being prepared for this should ease untoward reactions on the part of the therapists. Besides, these members add energy to a group that might otherwise be lacking, and they can be counted on to keep things moving along.

Unusual Group Members

The most difficult members to work with and those who may be most disruptive to the group include patients with transient cognitive disturbances caused by disease that has metastasis to the brain, those with lower IQ, and those with loosening of associations resulting from medication or generalized fatigue. Also difficult are those with disordered personality structure and members with extreme denial.

Cognitive Deficit

As a result of fatigue, medication, or brain involvement, some members may tend to dissociate away from current time, place, and logical sequence. They may occasionally ramble without a sense of purpose. If the member is not too disruptive and it appears that she can benefit from the group, supporting her constructive participation is important. The best way to manage such a member is to enter into an interactive dialogue with her for a minute or two and then to summarize and redirect to the group as a whole. This will help the member stay on track, show the member and the group that you care about what she is saying, and ease the worry of the group that this person will disrupt the group. When the patient is rambling on and on, therapists will have to interrupt politely (leaning forward, putting a hand out to get their attention, and saying "excuse me, I want to make sure I understand what you've been saying"), then briefly summarizing, perhaps asking them a concrete question, followed by redirecting to the group.

Personality Difficulties

Some members may come to the group with long-term personality characteristics that tend to disrupt the group. They may be

- interpersonally sensitive (socially avoidant or dependent) and afraid to speak their mind;
- interpersonally reactive (as with borderline personality qualities), needing yet afraid to get close to others;
- continually overwhelmed or especially emotionally demonstrative, crying out for attention (histrionic in nature);
- self-isolating or self-defeating, asking for help and then rejecting it; or
- needing to be the center of attention (with narcissistic tendencies) and to be seen by the group as the most important group member.

It is vital to form a liaison with the member. Not doing so will set up an uncomfortable battle within the group. Such a member is likely to have a much more complex interpretation of any interaction or lack of interaction. It is important to demonstrate an understanding of her feelings and thoughts through simple reflective listening, without reflection or interpretation. Having done this, it is useful to ask the group if this discussion has stimulated any thoughts or feelings about their own lives and situations. This approach helps to minimize the oversensitivity of these members to criticism or at least to limit their interference of the group.

However, therapists must be clear that this is not a group therapy for people with personality disorders; rather, the purpose is to aid adjustment to breast cancer. Therefore, reflecting on the personality characteristics of these members will rarely be of value to the group and may lead to conducting "individual therapy" inside the group or simply to alienating the member. If disruption continues, it may be necessary to speak with such members outside of the group about their special sensitivities or "insights" and ask for their assistance in allowing others to explore issues in their own way. If all else fails, it may be necessary to suggest to such members that a group format may not be the best type of support for them and that individual therapy may be of greater assistance.

Cognitive Avoidance or Emotional Repression

Some degree of avoidance and repression may be a buffer against excess distress (Dunkel-Schetter, Feinstein, & Taylor, 1992). However, problems arise when one always looks at the bright side of things, always keeps busy, and avoids anything to do with the cancer. In our experience with one group we facilitated, Betty was such a person. She did not want to discuss negative feelings or thoughts in the group, and she insisted on always telling others that they would be able to beat the cancer as long as they kept a positive attitude and did not let the cancer "get them down." Given that this was a group of recurrent cancer patients, they initially wanted to believe her view. After a few weeks, however, they heard how she would keep herself constantly busy to avoid having quiet reflective time in which "negative" thoughts might arise. She admitted to being so exhausted at the end of the day that she would be able to go immediately to sleep without any negative thoughts intruding. As soon as she awoke, she was up and working again. It was clear that Betty was becoming increasingly exhausted and that her quality of life was not a model that others wanted to emulate. After some time in the group, however, Betty was able to tolerate hearing other women discussing their fears and eventually to begin expressing her own fears. As a result, she was able to be calmer and more comfortably "in the moment," able to better enjoy each day of her remaining life. This was the Betty from whom other group members were able to learn and who they grew to respect.

Mood Disorders

Some degree of worry and sadness is to be expected and is even healthy. To not experience profound sadness or worry following a life-threatening diagnosis and life-shattering treatment would be bizarre. Yet, when a person clearly is manifesting the symptoms of depression or panic, serious attention must be paid to them. Certainly, a person with a serious panic or depressive disorder should be considered for referral. However, the group can assist many of these individuals, with or without the need for individual therapy (depending on the severity of their depression and their responsiveness to group treatment).

In the case of anxious depression, where the person is unable to sleep or concentrate because of intrusive thoughts, the group can help by giving reassurance, putting things in perspective, allowing the woman to express these worries rather than keep them continually inside, and practicing relaxation techniques. For those members who are experiencing a melancholic form of depression, the group can draw them out and help to give them realistic feedback for their cognitive distortions, boost their self-esteem, show them that others do care, and help them appreciate that there is much to live for. Those with dysthymic depression can benefit, perhaps osmotically, from the group's energy. Discussions of healthy lifestyle, such as exercise, healthy eating, and socializing, will also be a great service to these individuals.

People with anxiety disorders benefit tremendously from the group experience. The group will not raise issues that *cause* anxiety in breast cancer patients; rather, it serves to *express* those fears that cancer patients carry around with them on a regular basis. With the expression comes relief. Certainly, anxious patients may experience more manifest anxiety when first hearing and expressing issues related to their cancer. Yet with group support, seeing others tolerating these issues, and with the relaxation techniques that train their mind to focus on comfortable sensations in the moment, the group may be the best anxiolytic available for them.

Somatoform Disorders

Cancer patients are naturally worried about new feelings in their body, because it may indicate a progression of the disease. Some degree of somatic vigilance is certainly appropriate. However, group members not infrequently appear to express their distress through somatic means. One way to understand this phenomenon is to appreciate that people have to find some way to express their distress. Some individuals become anxious and have intrusive thoughts that make it difficult for them to sleep at night or concentrate during the day. Many people find themselves depressed or angry and blame others for their problems. Still others express their distress somatically. The benefit of this is that one feels comparatively stable, mentally, while their bodies take the brunt of the stress.

The somatoform disorders can manifest in various ways. Those with undifferentiated somatoform disorder or conversion disorder typically have low personal insight as well as low reflective ability. That is, they do not think much about their condition, yet they know that they hurt. They tend to externalize responsibility, expecting their doctors to find, explain, and treat their discomfort. For these people, focusing exclusively on active coping will lead to nothing but frustration. Instead, the model for these patients is the group's emphasis on discussion of problems and what they personally can do about them. If there is a good base of supportive rapport, therapists can occasionally ask nonthreatening questions about their personal, specific, and affective reaction to their problems and what they are doing actively to cope with the problem. Although they may respond in passive and externalizing terms, others are bound to jump in with personal and active suggestions. Eventually, a change may begin to occur.

In contrast, people with hypochondriasis or somatization disorders tend to have low personal insight yet tend toward excessive reflective moods. That is, they think too much about their condition, and in paying too much attention to their somatic sensations they enhance them. Some individuals are invested in being ill and derive tremendous benefit from it. Perhaps they relish the attention they receive from family and physicians. Perhaps it is an excuse not to function as fully as possible. Whatever the secondary gain, these individuals can benefit from the group in several ways. First, the regular weekly attention given to them will reduce unnecessary physician contacts. Being in a group of people with similar illnesses who are handling it well may serve as a useful model for their behavior. Learning to comfort oneself through the relaxation practice will be useful in redirecting attention from worry about somatic sensations to competitive comfortable sensations. The difficulty with these individuals is that they can be an energy drain for the group. It will be necessary for therapists to offer support, to ask them how they can react more optimally given their situation (perhaps, like others in the group), and then to redirect the discussion.

In all somatoform disorders (and in coping with pain for that matter), one common theme is to not overattend to somatic sensations. There are always competing sensations that are much more pleasant to attend to. Train the somatically focused individual to control her "reaction" to the pain and to control her "attention" to the pain (both of which serve to enhance her discomfort) by noticing when she is focused on the discomfort, and then attempt to focus on a more pleasant sensation or an activity. The meditation exercises in the Appendix are extremely useful for persons with somatoform disorders.

Terminating a Member's Participation

Although the group is encouraged to regulate itself through its own interactions, the ultimate responsibility for maintaining the frame rests with the therapists. The therapists must respond to any threat to the integrity and structure of the group and facilitate group discussion of these issues when necessary. It is helpful to remember that this is a time-limited group, and the devotion of disproportionate time and attention to the repetitive violations of a particular member of the group contract is not likely to help other members. Clear discussion with such a member of others' reactions to her behavior and the way it may be interfering with the needs of the group is likely to provide a positive model for working through other areas of conflict in group members' lives. In extreme cases, however, it may become clear that to protect the benefits of the group for others, a particular member's participation must be terminated. An argument can be made that in a much longer or open-ended group, it might be most helpful to allow the group to come to terms with this necessity over time and to participate more fully in such a decision. In this context, however, it is recommended that the therapists take final responsibility for making such a decision (in consultation with the supervising therapists) and that this be handled outside the group. There are generally a variety of responses to such an authoritarian action on the part of the therapists, including feelings in some members that may be strongly negative. It is important to allow expression of these feelings and to acknowledge openly the disadvantages of the course of action chosen.

Termination may also be chosen by a group member. Some may drop out because they expected something different from the group. Others may simply discover that they cannot devote the time and energy needed to attend. No amount of preparatory explanation or literature can correct all of these problems. However, good descriptive literature, pre-interviews, and adequate explanation at enrollment and at the first meeting of the purpose and style of the group and the time commitment required can help to minimize drop-outs. When a member does leave the group, it would be helpful if she can attend at least one more group session to explain her reasons for leaving the group and to say goodbye. This need not take up the entire session, but some time should be carved out to address the issue. If the patient does not wish to attend a final group session, then some time in the next session should still be devoted to addressing the loss of the member. Once again, an open and honest approach toward loss of any kind in the group helps group members address their own personal losses.

The Breast Cancer Notebook: Content and Therapeutic Issues

7

A companion patient volume, *The Breast Cancer Notebook: The Healing Power of Reflection* (Stanton & Reed, 2002), has been developed to assist cancer patients participating in group therapy to become more actively involved in coping with their cancer. Although the approach to group psychotherapy discussed here can certainly stand on its own, the use of *The Breast Cancer Notebook* is highly encouraged, especially with newly diagnosed patients. This chapter offers a brief overview of the notebook and suggests guidelines for successfully using it to enhance the benefits of group therapy.

Overview of The Breast Cancer Notebook

Purpose

The Breast Cancer Notebook contains 12 chapters as well as thought-provoking questions intended to assist patients to explore the impact that the cancer has on their lives and consider ways to more actively cope with and adjust to their new situation.

Although many therapeutic groups discuss important issues during sessions, it is unclear to what extent these issues continue to be worked on between sessions. *The Breast Cancer Notebook* is intended to enhance group therapy by encouraging participants to think about psychosocial issues relevant to their current life situation during the week. In addition, the notebook is meant to support group therapy by motivating patients to raise these issues during the group meetings. Thus, it offers a therapeutic bridge that extends from the therapy groups to the patients' lives and back to the group.

THERAPEUTIC CONSIDERATIONS

The Breast Cancer Notebook can be a valuable tool for both patient and therapist. Like any tool, however, it must be used with skill. There may be groups that require additional incentive to engage in meaningful discussion, in which case the exercises can serve as an excellent stimulus. On the other hand, patients who come prepared to discuss important issues relevant to their current life situation may feel constrained if they feel obliged to discuss a notebook chapter assigned by the therapists. Therefore, the therapists should pay particular attention at Check-In so that relevant and important patient issues are not superceded by text topics. For this reason, only the first few and the final chapters are intended to correspond to the first few and final group sessions. The therapists can suggest other chapters as particular topics arise naturally in the group.

FLEXIBLE STRUCTURE

The Breast Cancer Notebook also allows therapists to design a more or less structured group. For those inclined toward a more structured style of therapy, either because of group composition or therapist familiarity, each chapter of the notebook could correspond to a particular meeting of the group, with some chapters extending over two or more group sessions. Discussion could begin with patients' reactions to the chapter and the exercises it contains. Such structure may enhance the discussion of the specific topics covered in the chapter, but it also may tend to constrain more spontaneous discussion of issues of concern to patients. Therefore, as discussed above, the Check-In procedure takes on special importance for ensuring that personally relevant issues always take precedence over conceptually selected themes.

For therapists who choose to run a less structured group, the chapters can be assigned as needed. Each patient can decide for herself when a chapter may be relevant for her, or the therapists might recommend a chapter that becomes relevant as a result of emerging themes for any given group. In either case, patients should be encouraged to bring up thoughts and feelings that may be stimulated by *The Breast Cancer Notebook*. Therapists running a less structured group might even have participants consider an exercise in the middle of a group session to stimulate or focus a discussion. Whatever type of group therapists plan to conduct, the notebook should support their efforts.

In recommending the procedures described in chapter 4 for integrating *The Breast Cancer Notebook* with the group and for structuring the first few group sessions, we have attempted to strike what we believe to be an appropriate balance of structure. As noted, we encourage therapists to be attentive to the needs of their group members.

CHAPTERS

The first few chapters of *The Breast Cancer Notebook* have been designed to correspond to the first few group therapy meetings, as described in chapter 4, and address specific concerns common to almost all breast cancer patients. Similarly, the final chapter corresponds to the final group session. The other eight chapters can be selected by patients or therapists as they wish (see Exhibit 7.1).

Each chapter has a common structure:

▮ introduction to the topic,
▮ questions to ask oneself, and
▮ resources for further exploration of the topic.

The following is an outline of the chapters, with suggestions about some specific issues that therapists may address when introducing and discussing these topics. Therapists should also read the chapters themselves and think about what parts of the material may be most relevant for their group.

Finding Your Way

The introduction and first chapter explain the purpose of *The Breast Cancer Notebook*, along with the general layout and suggestions for use. The first chapter attempts to help women at various stages of disease and treatment to feel comfortable in their use of the text. The first chapter provides an extensive guide to cancer-related resources, including Web sites, books, and organizations.

EXHIBIT 7.1

Chapters in and Structure of *The Breast Cancer Notebook: The Healing Power of Reflection*

1. Finding Your Way
2. How Are You Coping With Breast Cancer?
3. Breast Cancer Treatment
4. Coping With Side Effects
5. Communicating With Members of Your Medical Team
6. Family and Friends
7. Work
8. Body Image and Sexuality
9. Feeling Better: Relaxation, Nutrition, and Exercise
10. Ending Treatment
11. Suggestions for the Soul
12. Finishing the Group

Psychotherapeutic considerations: Each group member will have questions and concerns about entering the group. If group members have reviewed *The Breast Cancer Notebook* in advance, they may have an impression that the group is more information oriented than psychotherapy oriented. Therefore, therapists are encouraged to make special effort to explain the nature of the group meetings and focus the discussions on patients' expressions rather than provide information.

How Are You Coping With Breast Cancer?

The second chapter begins by asking group members to consider how they are responding to what is happening to them. This chapter attempts to normalize many of the thoughts and feelings women may have by discussing common reactions among cancer patients. These include a sense of loss, fears about death, and difficulties in understanding and expressing such feelings. The popular belief about entertaining positive thoughts to the exclusion of negative thoughts and feelings is also addressed. Group members are encouraged to express as much or as little as they wish in the therapy sessions, which allows at least some measure of control over this aspect of the cancer experience.

The questions at the end of the chapter relate to group members' experience of stress, coping techniques that helped them in the past, and new ways of coping they may be exploring as they adapt to their breast cancer experience. Other questions explore how coping with past challenges affects their response to current challenges. Group members are also given a checklist intended to help them to identify their emotional and cognitive states. Resources for further exploration of the topic are included.

Psychotherapeutic considerations: Chapter 2 is intended to correspond to Group Session 2, during which patients are asked to "tell their stories." The chapter facilitates group members' focusing on their reactions to events rather than merely describing the events. However, some patients may be reluctant to delve into or reveal intimate thoughts and feelings in the initial group meetings. They may have no history of expressing personal thoughts or feelings to relative strangers or in public; they may believe that it is a sign of weakness to talk about personal problems; or they may feel overwhelmed with the diagnosis, treatment, or other events occurring in their lives. Therefore, although therapists should certainly ask about patients' reactions to events, they should respect patients' hesitancy to reveal such feelings. In addition, some patients may not have read *The Breast Cancer Notebook* chapter or answered the questions. No pressure should be brought to bear on these patients, because they may have many important things going on in their lives at the moment, and the group session should feel like a relief rather than an additional burden. Those who have used the book, however, may serve as models for stimulating the discussion along meaningful lines.

Breast Cancer Treatment

Chapter 3 helps patients focus on their responses to breast cancer treatment they have been or will be receiving. The chapter focuses on patients' experiences and ways of coping with treatment. It acknowledges the importance of treatment information and assists patients in formulating questions to ask their doctors. As with the other chapters, an effort is made to help normalize typical experiences and reactions during treatment. Common concerns addressed include how women feel about the treatment they are receiving and their thoughts about alternative or complementary treatments.

Questions focus on helping patients understand the treatment they may be undergoing, treatment side effects, and recommendations from their physicians for alleviating symptoms. Group members are prompted to explore other strategies for coping with treatment or to describe solutions they may have that might be useful to others. Separate sets of questions for exploration are included for women in treatment and those who have completed treatment. The resources at the end of this chapter offers, among other things, books written by and about women undergoing breast cancer treatment.

Psychotherapeutic considerations: This chapter is intended to correspond to Group Session 3. It should help women share their common experiences with breast cancer treatment in hopes that it will help normalize their difficulties and encourage them to communicate more effectively with their health care providers. In addition, the difficult question of alternative and complementary approaches is addressed early on, which lets patients know that they can feel free to talk about any issues that are important to them. In this meeting, as well as all future meetings, patients will be encouraged to relate not only their difficulties but also their successes, sharing coping strategies that have proven effective for them.

Patients should be cautious when sharing personal values and experiences. Those who truly believe in a particular approach (be it prayer, a book, an alternative medicine, or a relaxation technique) tend to foist it rather imperiously on others. These individuals generally do this out of a desire to be helpful and a conviction that their approach can benefit others. Therapists must walk a tightrope between acknowledging the benefits the individual has experienced and supporting her efforts at coping, on the one hand, and being clear that each person must find what works best for herself, on the other. No single approach—whether a treatment or a self-help technique—will work for all patients. The group is a useful place to share what each person has experienced to provide for more options. Hence, therapists should be concerned when a patient is more interested in proselytizing an approach to others than in using the group to explore other ways of coping. A simple yet effective approach to such individuals is to ask them to give a specific example of how the method they recommend has helped them in their lives (i.e., asking them to give specific personal examples).

Coping With Side Effects

As described in chapter 4 of this book, we recommend that Group Session 4 be less structured such that the correspondence between this chapter and the fourth session may be less visible. Although some treatment side effects are addressed in chapter 3, this chapter more fully explores self-help techniques and body changes. It begins by normalizing the temporary and permanent physical changes resulting from treatment (ranging from mastectomy to hair loss) and then turns to psychophysical (weight, fatigue, nausea) and psychological changes (mood). Anxiety over upcoming chemotherapy and radiation appointments is also addressed. This chapter also raises the issue of breast reconstruction and prosthesis. Finally, permission to take care of oneself is discussed.

Questions are posed about physical and emotional reactions to treatment side effects and whether women have questions they might ask their doctors. As with the other chapters, separate sections present questions for contemplation by women in treatment and those who have completed treatment.

Psychotherapeutic considerations: Any group discussion of cancer treatment or its side effects in the group tends to lead to talking about cancer treatments in general. To steer away from abstract medical discussions, it is useful for therapists to keep patients focused on personal reactions to treatment and helpful coping strategies. Patients' insistence on discussing the latest treatments or medicines to relieve unwanted side effects can be an opportunity to promote improved communication between patients and their doctors. In addition, it will be useful to remind patients that a medication or technique that helps one person may have no effect for another, but there is usually some way that a patient can better cope with their treatment or treatment sequelae.

Communicating With Members of Your Medical Team

By the time the group reaches Session 5, there has already been considerable exploration of treatments or managing side effects. Chapter 5 takes the discussion further by focusing specifically on styles of communication and comfort in discussing important issues with one's doctors. This chapter begins by acknowledging the central role that doctors play in a cancer patient's life. It normalizes for them the plethora of questions that must arise for somebody in this situation and encourages patients to write down questions as they occur. Second opinions are also discussed with suggested ways to broach the subject with one's oncologist. Special considerations for women who have completed treatment or who have recurrent cancer are also presented.

Questions for self-exploration include appreciating what level of information each woman desires, the degree of choice she prefers regarding her treatment, and the degree of dialogue she wishes to have with her medical team. Patients are asked to list the names of their treatment team members and to record in a diary the questions they have for each member of the team. Exercises are also included to help group members practice communicating different messages to their physicians, including asking for second opinions when appropriate. Finally, group members are asked to reflect on any communication difficulties they may be having with members of their medical team and to imagine a more ideal interchange.

Psychotherapeutic considerations: This chapter offers an excellent opportunity for patients to discuss communication skills in general and their relationship with their doctors in particular. Frustrations are bound to arise when one patient talks about how wonderful her doctor is while another patient is less than enthusiastic about hers. The group usually serves as a wonderful resource for exploring ways of communicating more effectively one's needs and desires with the medical team. Therapists can even ask patients to role-play healthy, open, and assertive communication styles with each other. Occasionally, even role-playing passive-compliant or aggressive-insistent styles can be fun and informative. The communication skills learned here clearly extend to other areas of patients' lives in which improved communication would be beneficial.

Family and Friends

Chapter 6, which focuses on the important topic of family and friends, comes at a time when the group typically is forming strong bonds with each other. It is useful to have a discussion of changing relationships in one's life as the group forms increasingly supportive bonds. Family relationships are often taken for granted, and casual relations are frequently given even less consideration. Yet all that changes when one faces a life-threatening illness. Many issues are suddenly thrust on a woman facing breast cancer. These include how much to confide in family, friends, and acquaintances and the sometimes tricky balance between attending to one' own needs and attending to the needs of others. This chapter considers focusing on one's own personal needs; the tendency to want to protect others; issues that arise between partners; communication with parents, siblings, and other extended family members; and relating to acquaintances and work associates. Other issues include concerns about passing along a breast cancer gene to daughters and questions about genetic testing. Finally, a good deal of consideration is given to communicating about one's disease with one's children.

Group members can be asked to list important persons in their lives, separately listing family members, friends, and coworkers, and to describe their relationship with these people and the benefits and the costs of these relationships in terms of their energy level and overall quality of life. Finally, group members are asked to reflect on ways that important relationships have changed since their cancer diagnosis and on ways that these relationships could be improved. An extensive list of further references is offered for patient exploration.

Psychotherapeutic considerations: This chapter relates to what can be one of the most important and surprisingly contentious topics for the group. Few things are so precious as one's family, and each woman has a different threshold about how much to reveal and to whom. As with all topics discussed in the group, diversity must be respected. Yet therapeutic intuition and scientific evidence point to the benefits of being able to openly and honestly express one's innermost thoughts and feelings to an intimate few. The desire to protect those closest to us, although noble, can often result in harm to ourselves and those we most desire to protect. Although no one would choose to develop breast cancer, many women report that they have become closer to their family and feel more rewards from that intimacy than they had ever imagined possible. On the other hand, some women in the group may require assistance in setting appropriate boundaries where colleagues or casual acquaintances are concerned. It is natural for acquaintances to want to help, but there are times when not saying "no" to unwanted help can increase overall distress. This is an opportunity to re-examine unwanted relationships as well as relationships that warrant further development.

Special consideration should be made for those who are single, have few friends, or are estranged from their family of origin. The issues need not be avoided, but instead therapists can ask directly of these individuals how they feel about the discussion regarding family and friends and what the patient might do to reduce their feelings of loneliness. It is important to be aware that, for some women, the group may offer the only close relationship they have.

Work

Chapter 7 addresses the range of work-related issues. Feelings of worth are associated with work, whether in the home or in a workplace. Workplace environments can range from being supportive to being stressful. Many women who have been self-reliant or have worked for others their whole lives may find it difficult to delegate responsibilities to others. Some women feel guilty taking time away from work. There are financial considerations, especially for women who are self-employed. Yet every woman with breast cancer must address serious and complicated financial arrangements whether that be employee or health insurance benefits or drawing on personal savings. Those who return to the workplace after completing their treatment or who look for new jobs have a unique set of circumstances to contend with, including whether or not to reveal their medical histories.

Questions for self-evaluation include reflecting on the most stressful and rewarding aspects of one's job before, during, and after the cancer diagnosis and treatment. What could be changed about one's work or one's attitude toward work to improve one's situation? How can one delegate parts of one's work to others? How does one feel about such delegation?

Psychotherapeutic considerations: Much of a person's identity and feeling of self-worth stem from her work, and discussion of work-related issues often leads to reflection about personal self-worth, self-efficacy in general, and other existential considerations. Many patients report feeling trapped by their need to work to earn a living. Other patients are trapped by their habit of working and their fear of having nothing to do if they take time off or retire early. This is further complicated by many patients' fear of "giving-in" to the cancer if they quit work. Once again, the group is an ideal environment for working out these issues. Those who have taken time off, retired, or merely allocated responsibility to others for a time can share their experiences with those who are contemplating similar actions. This chapter (and the next) can also stimulate exploration of fundamental existential issues.

Body Image and Sexuality

Body image issues were to some extent addressed earlier in the chapter on side effects; more enduring aspects of how breast cancer patients see themselves after the changes wrought by the cancer and treatment are more fully addressed in chapter 8. This chapter begins with a consideration of the image women have of their bodies, caring for their bodies, revealing their bodies, and going out in public. Issues of sexuality are addressed directly, including decreases in sexual pleasure and sexual desire and changes in sexuality across the breast cancer continuum. Issues of body image in sexuality are considered for single women, those in relationships, and those in stable partnerships.

Questions for self-evaluation include how one's body looks and feels to oneself and the changing experience of sexual pleasure before and after the breast cancer diagnosis. Also considered are the effects of changes in one's body image and sexuality for one's partner.

Psychotherapeutic considerations: Most women, especially those raised in American society, pay attention to how they look. The sudden radical changes that occur following breast cancer treatment (e.g., mastectomy, menopause, loss of hair, vaginal dryness) can strike a serious blow to women's fundamental sense of femininity. Many women report "feeling neutered" because of the treatment. This experience again can serve to help the group reflect on who they really are underneath their appearance. "What remains once these body changes take place?" "Who am I apart from my body?" Issues of sexuality are also complex. A woman might come back from surgery or chemotherapy feeling anything but sexual. Her partner may naturally be reticent to make sexual advances, and she might misinterpret this hesitancy as loss of sexual appeal. It is easy to understand how sexuality becomes downgraded in importance in the relationship. Couples often struggle with open discussion of sexual issues. Women rarely bring up these issues in group therapy unless prompted to do so. Therefore, therapists must feel comfortable about openly addressing issues of body image and sexuality to be able to support group members in expressing themselves on this important aspect of their lives. Group members may need substantial support to take the first step in letting their partners know about their desires for intimacy. In addition, the importance of intimacy in all forms should be supported.

Feeling Better: Relaxation, Nutrition, and Exercise

As described, each group session should contain a relaxation component (Opening and Closing Relaxations). Chapter 9 expands on this by focusing on a variety of healthy lifestyle activities. Recommendations for improving self-comfort, sleep, diet, and exercise are provided. Care is taken to allow for each patient to find the level of activity that is most effective for her individual situation. Specific recommendations for eating during and after oncotherapy are discussed.

Questions for self-evaluation include how effective the group relaxation exercises have been for the patient and how women might modify the exercises to suit their personal needs. Women also have an opportunity to examine their sleep patterns and consider ways to ameliorate any deficits. Finally, questions regarding diet and exercise as well as resources for pursuing these topics are presented.

Psychotherapeutic considerations: Patients undergoing cancer treatment rarely feel like exercising or worrying about eating healthfully. However, experience suggests that if they keep their calories up during treatment, engage in some exercise every day, and attempt to focus on soothing feelings, they can better tolerate their treatments. Therapists may remind them that few people feel like exercising, eating, or taking time to do a relaxation exercise during cancer treatments but that if they do these activities, despite their nausea or fatigue, they will probably find themselves feeling better. On the other hand, some women may find that they try too much or are too hard on themselves and must be given permission to take small steps until they find out how they are reacting to their new situation. Women who have completed treatment should be similarly urged to improve their quality of life through healthy lifestyle activities. Yet they also need to take small steps before returning to a level of activity they may have previously reached. Still other women have never exercised or focused on what they eat, and self-help relaxation exercises are completely new for them. Therefore, as in all material covered in the groups, a wide variety of attitudes and approaches to healthy lifestyle must be expected and tolerated.

Ending Cancer Treatment

Chapter 10 may be most important for women who are currently receiving treatment or who have finished treatment recently. The chapter addresses strong feelings that typically arise at the end of cancer treatment. These include a great sense of relief as well as a deep fear: "Now that I am finished with treatment, does that mean the cancer is gone, or that there's nothing more that can be done for me? Am I still a cancer patient, or have I recovered from cancer?" Now begins the wait for the magical "5-year" mark, when it is less likely that the cancer will recur. There are many reminders of the cancer, including follow-up visits, anniversaries, and fears of recurrence that may be experienced with every minor pain or small change in energy level. Positive issues arise at this juncture as well, including feeling that it is time to move on or feeling that this is a beginning instead of an end. Finally, the termination of treatment can be an impetus for establishing new priorities and goals for the rest of one's life.

Questions for self-evaluation include what one is feeling physically and emotionally at the end of treatment. There may be a disconnect between how a woman feels and how those around her view her. Expectations about work may require re-evaluation. Questions regarding loss and confusion as well as a new sense of self are posed. The possibilities of reordering priorities and committing to aspects of one's life that will bring greater meaning and value are offered for self-reflection.

Psychotherapeutic considerations: Many cancer researchers and therapists have found that patients are much more likely to address existential aspects of their life in the shadow of cancer when treatment ends. Up to this point patients are struggling to get through each day. At the end of treatment, however, they often experience a sort of "let down" in which the struggle to keep up can subside and thoughts and feelings that have been pushed down for many months now begin to surface. It is also at this time that patients begin to look toward the future and what the future might hold for them both quantitatively and qualitatively. In other words, patients experiencing the end of treatment while in the group can benefit greatly when therapists recognize this time as a potentially important time in their growth and development.

Suggestions for the Soul

Not everyone believes in an all-powerful deity or attends an organized church. Yet every person knows what it means to feel more or less at peace, integrated in mind, body, and spirit. It is often difficult to regain a sense of well-being after a long period of trauma. Chapter 11 helps patients to find activities that bring them greater sense of harmony and an integrated sense of peace and well-being. Patients are encouraged to make time for themselves, find quiet time on a regular basis, discover new ways to laugh, and eliminate stressors.

Questions for self-examination include considering future activities that will bring a greater sense of meaning, purpose, and value to life. These questions are intended to assist group members in finding ways to eliminate stress and discover ways of feeling better. Resources are offered on subjects such as reducing anxiety, relaxing, and discovering the life transitions of others who have had cancer and the value of personal expression.

Psychotherapeutic considerations: Some patients will find new commitment and comfort in their lifelong religion. Others will find such comfort in seemingly little things, such as a walk in the park, playing with their children or grandchildren, or snuggling up with a good book in front of a fire. The benefit of the group is found in the richness of individual experience that allows each woman to find the path to a greater sense of harmony. It is this sense of harmony that therapists can help the group appreciate rather than any particular activity from which it is generated. Such an attitude will help prevent individuals from proselytizing and can help each member focus on what is important in her life.

Finishing the Group

Chapter 12 is intended to correspond to the last session or last couple of sessions of the psychotherapy group. Group termination arouses considerable uncertainty and a sense of ambiguity. On the one hand, patients may be openly relieved to be ending this phase of their lives. On the other hand, there have been many important intrapersonal and interpersonal developments in the course of group therapy that patients are generally reluctant to let go. Toward this end, patients' feelings about the ending of the group are normalized. They may feel that there is still much unfinished business to attend to and that they have accomplished many things during the group sessions, and they may have considerable sadness at saying goodbye to their friends in the group.

Experiential exercises include journaling one's impressions of others in the group and changes they have undergone throughout the course of therapy. Feelings about the group and finished and unfinished business are also considered, as well as strategies for continuing to work on some of the processes begun in the group.

Psychotherapeutic considerations: This topic is important not only in that it assists in bringing closure to the group, but also because it serves as a metaphor for transitioning from struggling with cancer to a new phase in the patient's life. The way that group termination is handled will assist group members in more openly and comfortably addressing issues of termination in their lives, whether that be letting go of old habits, activities, and relationships or coming to terms with their own mortality. The group can be considered not only a supportive environment to buffer one's distress but also as training that assists patients in living as fully as possible from this point forward. Issues of termination should therefore be addressed sooner than the last session, and the time-limited nature of the group should be kept in mind throughout.

At least once in the middle of the series of group therapy sessions and probably again toward the end, it is useful to revisit the topic of the second notebook chapter: taking stock of how patients are coping. Certainly the Check-Ins address this issue to some extent at each session. However, focusing on how their ability to cope has changed over the course of therapy can be a useful exercise for group members. In addition, it can be useful to reflect on how the group is going for them and perhaps on some directions they have yet to explore.

Psychotherapeutic considerations: Because this is a more supportive than exploratory form of psychotherapy, the therapist should not spend too much time discussing group process issues. However, some degree of reflection on where the patient has been and where she would like to go with regard to the group is very beneficial. Such reflection helps patients feel that they are to some extent in control of the group, as well as help them take responsibility for their own changes.

Final Thoughts

The Breast Cancer Notebook can greatly facilitate both individual and group processes, although we do not see it as a mandatory part of the group therapy model presented in this book. It allows patients both to prepare for upcoming groups as well as continue to reflect on issues that have arisen in the groups. Therapists new to this process or those who are working with a group that tends to be more passive may find that assigning specific chapters for specific meetings throughout the group is helpful. For therapists who wish to run groups without a predetermined schedule of topics, using the first few chapters to correspond to the first several sessions of therapy can facilitate patients' involvement in the group and contribute to the development of group cohesiveness. Group members can then select chapters that correspond to their particular needs or interests, or therapists can select them in response to issues that have emerged in the group. *The Breast Cancer Notebook* also becomes a diary of group members' experiences with cancer and a method of reexamining various aspects of their coping with cancer throughout their lives.

Other Types of Groups, Other Types of Cancer, and Other Settings

8

Although the approach described in the preceding chapters is primarily for use in groups of women with breast cancer, we have used a very similar approach with groups of patients with a variety of medical illnesses. We now describe indications for use of this same approach as well as ways to modify this approach in other populations.

Different Approaches for Different Types of Groups

The approach discussed thus far can be readily modified for use with different patient populations. Therapeutic emphasis can vary depending on the stage of illness, type of illness, and the extent to which the groups comprise similar or dissimilar members.

HOMOGENOUS VS. HETEROGENEOUS GROUPS

Compared with groups whose members have various illnesses, it is generally far easier to facilitate a group of people who have the same diagnosis and are at the same stage of disease progression. If group members are similar in age and gender, they generally have more in common, the group will be more cohesive and the discussions deeper, all of which make the therapists' job far easier. A group of single women younger than 40 with a first occurrence of breast cancer have many special concerns in common that they would be able to address during the group. In contrast, the most difficult type of group to facilitate is one in which there are a dozen members of varying ages and both genders, each with a different medical illness and at varying stages of disease progression. Although the type of homogenous group described above is typically only feasible in a specialized cancer center because of recruitment issues, the point is that patients more readily benefit from groups containing people most similar to themselves.

Because highly homogenous groups are often impractical to recruit, we describe heterogeneous groups as well. In general, the more heterogeneous a group, the harder the therapists must work to pull for commonalities and interactions among group members, which more naturally arise in the homogenous groups. Therefore, the more heterogeneous a group, the more active the therapists become, and the more structured the group must be (in terms of, e.g., structured exercises that emphasize common themes, check-ins, check-outs).

DIFFERENT STYLES OF FACILITATION

As discussed in chapter 3, various therapeutic styles are required to meet the needs of various types of patients. When the goal of the group is to disseminate knowledge, as in prevention-oriented groups, a deductive teaching style is indicated. When the group's purpose is to develop coping skills (e.g., in the case of patients newly diagnosed with a life-threatening illness), an interactive cognitive–behavioral approach with some teaching and open discussion is common. However, the inductive approach described in this book appears to be most effective for patients learning to live with a chronic life-threatening illness (see Table 8.1).

PATIENTS WITH VARIOUS STAGES OF ILLNESS

Deciding which approach to take is best determined by the needs of the patients. These needs can best be understood by examining the issues that arise at various stages of illness. As described in Table 8.2, women at different stages of breast cancer have differing issues they wish to address and goals to attain. Therapists need to adjust the methods and structure of therapy to accommodate them. Several examples are offered below. These examples are gleaned from our own clinical experience as well as from the experience of therapists who have reported success with this approach in the research literature. These principles seem to apply equally across all types of cancer (and many other life-threatening illnesses, for that matter).

Prevention

Cancer patients who are at increased risk for disease incidence or recurrence often benefit from education about preventive measures. Yet

TABLE 8.1

Therapeutic Style Differs by Group Structure and Goals

Goals of group	Therapeutic style		
	Deductive	Interactive	Inductive
Information, knowledge	X	x	—
Coping skills	x	X	x
Social and emotional support	—	x	X

Note. An X indicates primary therapeutic emphasis, an x indicates minor emphasis, and a dash indicates negligible emphasis. From "Group Therapy for Persons with Cancer," by J. Spira, in *Psychooncology* (p. 709), edited by J. Holland, 1998, New York: Oxford University Press. Copyright 1998 by Oxford University Press. Reprinted by permission.

some discussion of stress and stress management is helpful as well. The method of education is didactic, most often in a brief format (between one and six weekly meetings). Although the teaching process is primarily deductive, the more interactive the educational process (with questions from the group and discussion among group attendees), the better the material is learned and applied.

Diagnosis

Patients who have recently received an initial diagnosis of cancer are naturally distressed over the diagnosis and are no doubt confused about cancer and its etiology, treatment, and prognosis. Patients at this stage may benefit from basic education about stress management, to reduce anxiety and cope with immediate decisions regarding treatment, and emotional support. Although some deductive intervention is useful for offering basic information, therapeutic facilitation is primarily interactive for developing active coping skills, with some inductive facilitation for supportive discussion. It is difficult to mix didactic and interactive formats, because once they have been lectured to, patients find it difficult to switch to a group discussion or format with any real depth of emotional expression. Therefore, many therapists find it beneficial to separate the didactic education from the interactive components. Different meetings, different parts of meetings separated by a break, or even different facilitators can help patients to get the most out of each type of method. The number of group sessions is typically small, allowing for drop-ins to accommodate those who just received a diagnosis and are about to undergo surgery and other time-consuming treatments. Unfortunately, these types of groups are rarely offered, perhaps because patients are too consumed with the sudden change of their

TABLE 8.2

Therapeutic Goals, Methods, and Structures Useful For Addressing the Special Issues of Specific Cancer Populations

Stage of illness	Special issues	Goals	Methods	Structure
Prevention	At increased risk for disease incidence or recurrence	Education	Deductive: didactic information	Brief class (1–4 meetings)
Diagnosis	Distress over diagnosis Confusion about cancer	Education Coping in moment Emotional support	Interactive: ■ didactic information ■ experiential skills Inductive: supportive discussion	Brief group (1–6 weeks)
Treatment	Discomfort: nausea, mucus membranes, fatigue, weight Reality of illness sets in	Coping with treatment Adjusting one's life to having cancer Emotional support	Interactive: experiential skills Inductive: supportive discussion	Brief group (4–12 weeks)
Recovery	Self-image (cancer patient?) Questioning life activities Relationships Sense of control Possible recurrence or death Attitudes and behavior affecting health	Active coping Emotional–social support Re-examining life values, beliefs, priorities Considering one's future Living a healthy lifestyle	Interactive: ■ cognitive therapy ■ experiential skills Inductive: supportive discussion	Short-term (8–16 weeks)

Recurrence and dying	Emotional distress Death and dying Coping with treatment Loss of control Family and friends Physical discomfort or fatigue	Active coping Pain and stress management Emotional and social support Existential issues Living fully in the moment	Inductive: supportive discussion Interactive: experiential skills	Long term (24 weeks–ongoing)
Family members and bereavement	Emotional distress Existential issues Guilt	Emotional support Work through distress Living more in the moment Planning for the future	Inductive: supportive discussion Interactive: experiential skills	As needed: ▪ brief formats, support persons attend with patients ▪ longer formats, support and bereaved members meet separately

Note. From "Group Therapy for Persons with Cancer," by J. Spira, in *Psychooncology* (p. 712), edited by J. Holland, 1998, New York: Oxford University Press. Copyright 1998 by Oxford University Press. Reprinted by permission.

circumstances and beginning oncotherapy to fit in another, "less vital" treatment. Nonetheless, when offered, this type of group is of tremendous value for the newly diagnosed patient. It can also serve as a transitional group, in which patients can begin therapy and then, when they are more stable in their lives and treatment regimes, move on to a more committed group. Frequently, groups held for cancer patients immediately following diagnosis or for those in the early stages of treatment are those in which the group is presented as part of the cancer treatment.

Treatment

Special issues for people undergoing treatment may include the need to deal with recovery from surgery and discomfort from chemotherapy and radiotherapy, which often includes fatigue, nausea, dry or sore mucus membranes, weight changes, flulike symptoms, and so on. Changes in appearance (e.g., hair loss) and daily functioning are also common. With these changes occurring, the urgency of dealing with the initial diagnosis and treatment decisions passing, and the initial shock subsiding, the reality of the illness begins to set-in. Patients at this stage are concerned with coping with treatment, adjusting to life as a cancer patient, and receiving emotional support. An interactive therapeutic style that offers emotional support, discussion of healthy lifestyle, and experiential coping skills is therefore appropriate and can be delivered effectively for most patients in a brief (4–12 weeks) group, at least initially. Although these groups operate best if patients commit to attend all the sessions, patients are often allowed to begin at any time to accommodate those just beginning treatment. Also, patients in treatment frequently miss groups to accommodate changing treatment schedules as well as severe treatment reactions. Therefore, a rotating schedule of topics is helpful. Although groups for newly diagnosed patients or for those in treatment should be offered, most cancer patients are so occupied with their treatments that they do not become interested in group therapy until they are close to ending or completely finished with treatment. Again, however, if the group is presented as part of their total treatment, as a way to better tolerate their oncotherapy and maintain a higher level of quality of life, patients are more likely to participate.

Recovery

When patients complete treatment for an initial occurrence of cancer, their concern is to return to a normal life. They become interested in discussing changes in self-image ("Am I a cancer patient?) and changes in relationships, questioning and reprioritizing daily activities, wanting more control over their health and course of disease, wondering whether personality or behavior affects their health, and considering the possibility of disease recurrence and death. The therapeutic goals for this stage include training patients in active coping strategies; offering emotional and social support; reexamining life values, beliefs, and priorities; and learning to live a mentally and physically healthy lifestyle. An interactive therapeutic method, based on an inductive facilitation of supportive discussion, along with some structured exercises and teaching experiential relaxation skills, helps achieve these goals, usually in a short-term (8–16 weeks) group format. The type of therapy described in this book is adequate for this population, especially in combination with *The Breast Cancer Notebook: The Healing Power of Reflection* (Stanton & Reed, 2002).

Recurrence and Dying

Patients who experience disease recurrence face substantial emotional distress (quite likely re-experiencing distress from the initial diagnosis plus the likelihood of dying within the next few years); protracted and intensive treatment; greater loss of control, physical discomfort, and fatigue; reduced daily functioning; decisions regarding retirement and disability; new ways of relating to family and friends; and also more direct confrontation of the likelihood of dying. Learning to cope more actively, managing pain and stress, receiving emotional support, addressing existential issues, and living more fully in each moment are all beneficial to patients at this stage of illness. An inductive approach allowing for supportive discussion and occasional facilitation of experiential skills (relaxation, self-hypnosis) can facilitate these goals in a longer format (16 weeks and beyond). The style of therapy described in this book works very well with this population, although much of *The Breast Cancer Notebook* will be redundant with these "expert" patients.

Family Members and Bereavement

Families of cancer patients should not be neglected. Assisting family members to cope goes a long way in supporting the patient. Family members experience many of the same issues as do patients. Therefore, a style of therapy similar to that of the patient is appropriate for them as well. In early stages of treatment (for patients confronting prevention, diagnosis, and possibly brief groups for coping with treatment), it is valuable to have family members present in the groups. However, for longer term groups (longer than 4 weeks), patients and family members are better served in separate groups, so that they can discuss their concerns and not worry about distressing one another. Resources permitting, it may be convenient to have patients and family members meet at the same time, in adjacent rooms. Of course, not all patients have family members who are in the area or who would attend such groups, and this lack of support should be addressed in the patient groups.

Family members of patients who have died face considerable emotional distress, existential considerations, and possibly guilt. Offering emotional support to work through distress and help them to live more fully in the moment and plan for the future requires an inductive, interactive format, along with teaching some experiential skills (relaxation, self-hypnosis). Family members who have been involved in family groups while the patient was alive should be invited to stay on in the group for as long as they like. The therapeutic style described in this book is very appropriate for use with family members. Depending on the stage of illness of the patient, family members may find *The Breast Cancer Notebook* to be helpful. Certainly the existential exercises and experiential practices (relaxation, meditation, self-hypnosis) are very relevant to family members of patients in the later stages of treatment or illness.

Women With Recurrent Breast Cancer

HOMOGENOUS GROUPS

Women with recurrent breast cancer receive the greatest benefit from a group composed exclusively of women who have recurrent disease. Women dealing with a first occurrence or a recurrence of breast cancer have much in common. Women with both early- and late-stage disease want to live as fully as possible in each moment, reduce mental and physical discomfort, enjoy relationships, adjust to the changing circumstances of their lives, and find life activities that are most meaningful to them. However, the degree of concern for various issues is often different, and these differences in emphasis suggest a benefit in different groups for different stages of disease.

Women with a first occurrence of breast cancer typically try to put the cancer behind them and attempt to regain as normal a lifestyle as possible. They are often concerned with such issues as prosthesis, dating, work, and other ways to "normalize" their lives. Although they may have existential concerns, their primary focus is on coping with discomfort and worrying about the future. Women with recurrent breast cancer cannot put the cancer behind them. It is a central part of their daily existence. At times they may not be actively taking chemotherapy or radiation, but such hiatuses are usually only temporary. Life will never be "normal" again for them, and because recurrence is almost always terminal, they have death and dying issues to confront. In this case, existential issues are central to their lives.

When the groups are mixed, women with earlier stage disease may feel reluctant to bring up issues of dating or sexuality when there is someone who just announced that the disease has spread to her lungs and that she will be undergoing a painful procedure to extract fluid from them to help her breathe easier. Likewise, women with recurrent disease may feel reluctant to bring up issues of preparing for death for fear of distressing women in the group trying to put the disease behind them. Both issues are important and should be expressed and discussed. When the groups are separated by first and recurrent disease, the women are more willing to bring up these issues and to explore them in depth (Exhibit 8.1).

Because of the intensity of these issues, therapists facilitating these groups typically intervene less often to get the topics back on track. There is an intensity to recurrent groups that ensures that content is rarely lacking. Nonetheless, therapists play an important role in keeping the expressive and interactive processes intact.

Patients in these groups have been dealing with the issues contained in *The Breast Cancer Notebook* for some time, and as such the educational information that it contains is not new to them. However, the questions and exercises may be as thought provoking for them as for those with a first occurrence (albeit bringing up different issues to discuss).

Although groups of women with a first occurrence of breast cancer run the risk of identifying themselves as "cancer patients" and not moving beyond their cancer experience, women with recurrent breast cancer are in fact cancer patients, for the most part in treatment and facing their cancer on a daily basis. Therefore, ongoing groups are most effective for this population. It is nonetheless helpful to ask for a minimum

---

EXHIBIT 8.1

Issues Likely to Be Raised in Recurrent Breast Cancer Groups

There are several issues for women with recurrent disease that do not arise as frequently in groups for women with first occurrence, including

- bad news (metastasis, lack of responsiveness to treatment);
- death of a member (funerals, grieving in group);
- severe treatments requiring prolonged hospitalization;
- missing important future events of family members; and
- other issues relating to severity of disease, severity of treatment, and imminent loss of life.

commitment (say, 16 weeks) before deciding to recommit to the next 16 weeks. Unless therapists are recruiting patients from a large cancer treatment facility where they can recruit a new group of 8–12 women every month or two, starting new groups on such a regular basis is impossible. We suggest that to maintain the required numbers, new members be allowed to join on regular starting dates (for instance, the beginning of each month or every even month). This allows women in need to receive the benefit of the group, while at the same time minimizing group disruption. (In fact, this usually serves to stimulate discussion.) There will always be some "newcomer syndrome," with newly admitted members requiring a period of adjustment, but this will quickly change as still newer members are admitted to the group.

HETEROGENEOUS GROUPS

Where it is not feasible to conduct separate groups (usually because of the difficulty in recruiting a sufficient number of participants), mixed groups of first-occurrence and recurrent breast cancer patients are possible. However, because of the differences in issues between the two populations, mixed groups are extremely difficult to facilitate. Still, with skilled therapists, it is usually more valuable to patients to be part of a mixed-stage group than not to have a group at all.

Strategies for facilitating such groups include

- looking for commonalities;
- being up front about the differences in issues and how each is equally important to the people who have them (members need to express their concerns openly); and
- addressing the fear factor that recurrent issues bring up for those with a first occurrence of the disease.

In light of these factors, therapists may consider having a mixed type of cancer, all with similar stages of disease, rather than a mixed breast cancer group. This decision will be based on the interests and expertise of the therapists as well as on institutional factors (such as whether the therapists have been hired to facilitate only breast cancer groups). It is true that women with breast cancer have much in common and tend to more readily bond, even in a mixed-stage group. However, it often does not take long for members in a mixed-cancer or similar-stage group to form close relationships.

If a mixed group is formed because of recruitment limitations, one strategy is to conduct a mixed group for the first 16 weeks (using the protocol described in this book) and then ending the group for women with a first occurrence of breast cancer and enrolling the women with recurrent disease into an ongoing group exclusively for them. An alternate approach would be to have a combined coping-skills group for the first 8 weeks (using a more structured approach, more heavily relying on *The Breast Cancer Notebook*), and then having the first occurrence cancer women continue in an 8-week supportive-style group and the women with recurrent cancer merge with an ongoing long-term support group (based on the protocol used in this book).

People With Other Types of Cancer

We have used this approach, with some minor modifications, with patients with a variety of other forms of cancer and medical illnesses. Different types of cancer may suggest different types of groups.

GENDER-SPECIFIC CANCER

One way of organizing groups is by gender. Patients with gynecologic cancers or prostate cancer can be recruited to form groups. The gender specificity of the disease facilitates bonding due to commonalities among the disease and also gender-related issues.

Gynecologic-related cancers have in common all the issues discussed with breast cancer. In addition, they typically involve surgical mutilation of the genitalia and related sexual dysfunction. These cancers are less in the public eye and more embarrassing to discuss. Therefore, the type of group facilitation described in this book is optimal for this population. Many of the topics in *The Breast Cancer Notebook* can also apply. Although it is optimal to have separate groups for women at different stages of this cancer, its diagnosis is less common than breast cancer, so it may be necessary to facilitate a mixed-stage group.

Conducting a group for prostate cancer, on the other hand, requires considerable augmentation of the current format. Although similar to gynecological cancers in terms of gender and sexual dysfunction, special consideration should be given to the format because these groups are usually composed of older men. Typically, prostate cancer becomes "clinical" in an age group not known for emotional expression and for sharing of personal issues. Therefore, a more structured approach emphasizing a psychoeducational format is used for this population. The group typically begins with an educational review of a particular topic, followed by specific questions or an in-group exercise to explore this particular topic. This should generate enough interest and questions to begin an interactive discussion. However, because the group is so structured and the facilitator plays the role of content expert, most discussion is more often than not directed toward the facilitator. The therapist therefore must work extra hard to facilitate discussion among members. These groups also seem to work best when presented in a short-term format, typically 6 weeks. Of course, those men who wish to continue can recommit for an additional 6 weeks. Because prostate cancer groups are usually difficult to form, these groups most likely have men at mixed stages of their disease and concomitant mixed issues of concern.

MIXED-GENDER DISEASES

Lung cancer and colon cancer are other kinds of cancer for which this protocol is very useful. Colon cancer is similar to breast cancer in terms of staging and prognosis. Therefore, it is useful to separate the groups in terms of first-occurrence and recurrent disease whenever possible. Whereas breast cancer patients are concerned with mastectomy and possible prosthesis or reconstruction, many colon cancer patients have colostomies, which raise important issues that must be addressed directly.

Lung cancer has a more serious prognosis than most other common forms of cancer and therefore the next stage group is more appropriate. Even those who have been "successfully treated" have a very high risk of recurrent disease and subsequent death. In contrast to other forms of cancer, lung cancer is most frequently caused by smoking, a behavioral habit that therefore raises the issue of guilt for group members. Emphasis must be placed on taking responsibility for one's life now and in the future rather than dwelling on the past. The protocol as discussed in this book is highly applicable to the lung cancer population.

Leukemia among children and adolescents is a common disease that may warrant group therapy. The protocol discussed in this book is very effective when conducted for parents of children with leukemia. However, children's groups require a very different approach than that described above. First of all, it is extremely difficult, if not impossible, to conduct a single group for children ranging in age from early childhood to late adolescence. In fact, even a range of five years (say, from ages 8–13) contain children who have vastly different cognitive, emotional, and social concerns. Although groups for children with leukemia are extremely beneficial, it takes special pediatric therapy skills to conduct a worthwhile group for this population.

Groups for other types of cancer might be organized if there is sufficient patient interest. However, most other forms of cancer have insufficient numbers to justify conducting a group solely for individuals with that specific disease. Therefore, it is useful to consider how one would conduct a mixed cancer type group.

MIXED CANCER TYPE OR STAGE

Occasionally, homogenous groups are impossible to fill because of limitations in recruiting. In that case, it may be better to conduct a heterogeneous group than not to have a group at all. This clearly would depend on the experience and skill level of the therapists. The more heterogeneous a group, the more difficult to conduct. As discussed above (in the context of homogenous vs. heterogeneous stage breast cancer groups), the more varied the groups (type, stage, gender, age) the more varied the concerns of the group members and the more difficult the bonding among members becomes. Still, the group can be of value if therapists can

- look for and facilitate commonalities among group members and
- permit expression of individual concerns, even when others may not relate directly to them.

There are three types of heterogeneous cancer groups : (a) mixed types of cancer (following a first occurrence and following a recurrence), (b) mixed stages of cancer (with a single type of cancer), and (c) mixed stages and types of cancer. Groups with mixed types of cancer appear to work best for patients with recurrent cancers. Even though the original cancer site may vary, these patients all have a great deal in common, including treatment severity, illness severity, end-of-life issues, and constancy of illness. Groups where patients all have had a first occurrence yet vary in types of cancer also vary tremendously in terms of treatment issues, prognosis, quality of life during and after treatment, and other factors that make it difficult to find psychosocial commonalities among them.

The protocol described in this book can be useful for heterogeneous groups. As a general rule, the more heterogeneous the group, the more the therapists must rely on organization (e.g., structured exercises and increased therapeutic intervention) to keep the process on track. Unfortunately, specific psychoeducational material (e.g., that contained within *The Breast Cancer Notebook*) with a common relevance is more difficult to find. The check-ins become especially important, because at that time therapists can begin to identify common themes that can draw in other group members.

However, even more structure is usually required in mixed type or stage cancer groups. It is usually beneficial to have a predefined series of topics to explore. The therapists can decide in advance what typical common themes are of interest to most of the group members. Therapists can give homework assignments (much like those contained in *The Breast Cancer Notebook*) for the group members to reflect on during the week prior to meeting. During the next group meeting, following the relaxation exercise and the check-in, therapists can lead with specific structured questions to draw out members' concerns about the specific issue. This should generate a lively interactive discussion, which can then be facilitated in the usual way.

People With Other Life-threatening Illnesses

It is not the purpose of this book to describe in any detail how group therapy for a variety of medical illnesses can be conducted with beneficial outcomes. That has been done elsewhere (Spira, 1997b). The protocol discussed in this book can be used in treating other life-threatening illnesses as well. However, it will need to be modified to varying extents, depending on whether the disease being treated has a real rehabilitation component.

DISEASES WITH A LIFESTYLE REHABILITATION COMPONENT

Patients in cardiovascular, diabetes, or pulmonary rehabilitation programs can benefit from a combination of education about their disease, education about the value of a healthy lifestyle, and psychotherapy. The psychotherapy component of such rehabilitation programs include

- stress management;
- skills for coping with treatment, illness, and rehabilitation;
- strategies for complying with healthy lifestyle recommendations; and
- exploration of existential issues involved in adjusting to their new lifestyle (both the illness and the recovery from the illness).

The method of group facilitation described in chapter 5 will be of value in facilitating the *psychotherapeutic component* of such rehabilitation programs. However, cardiopulmonary patients with a terminal illness (e.g., congestive heart failure) will benefit from a group more closely based on method described in this book.

DISEASES WITHOUT A MAJOR LIFESTYLE REHABILITATION COMPONENT

Whereas the protocol described in chapter 5 of this book is of great value to the psychotherapeutic component of a rehabilitation program for people facing a life-threatening illness, the entire protocol can be followed closely when coordinating groups of patients diagnosed with a life-threatening illness that is not especially amenable to rehabilitation. Examples of populations with whom this protocol has been used with only minor modifications include patients with multiple sclerosis (MS) and HIV/AIDS. Although people diagnosed with these illnesses have much in common with breast cancer patients, there are some notable differences that must be taken into account when applying this protocol to these special populations.

MS is a progressive degenerative neurological disease that has many different courses. Some patients have mild symptoms for many years; others are suddenly struck with severe symptoms that may or may not temporarily remit. Both cognitive and neuromotor symptoms are of concern to these patients. Unlike patients with a first occurrence of breast cancer, who lead fairly functional lives once treatment has been completed, patients with MS are constantly struggling with diminished capacity for performing daily functions. Fatigue and depression are also common. When the current protocol is used for this population, it is recommended that the entire population be included in the group, no matter what their stage of progression. Because practically all patients with MS at some point progress in their disease, it is useful for those with slower progression to both support others as well as see how well the others are holding up. Fear of the unknown—and even worse, fear of the imagined—can be avoided by having all stages in the same group. We have found that the protocol described in this book works well. Developing a notebook for patients with MS would also be quite effective.

HIV/AIDS is similarly a progressive and debilitating illness. Because of the new medications available in industrialized countries, patients with HIV can be expected to live for many years. Like patients with MS, people with HIV/AIDS benefit from inclusion of the entire range of patients, no matter what their stage of illness. The protocol described in this book has been followed closely with this population (Reed & Stanton, 2002). However, separate groups can and probably should be formed, not on the basis of disease progression but rather on the subculture of the people with HIV. Seropositive gay men tend to be much more informed about their disease and bond far more readily in the group than other populations. Male and female intravenous drug users have issues that are unique to them as well, such that a great deal of the group must focus on drug use and rehabilitation issues. Nonaddicted heterosexual individuals, if available in sufficient numbers, may require their own group.

Depending on the comfort level and skill level of the therapists, if separate groups are not feasible because of recruitment difficulty, a combined group can be attempted. However, some of the issues having to do with the particular subcultures are so unique (especially the intravenous drug users) as to cast doubt on the potential value of a combined group. Similar in format to the mixed breast cancer groups, it may be beneficial to have a 16-week group (as described in this book) and allow members (especially those with symptoms) to recommit to additional 16-week groups. Although most of the issues in HIV are practically identical with those of breast cancer, they tend to vary in emphasis (with social stigma, sexuality, and body image taking a somewhat higher profile in HIV groups). The use of a participant notebook is also recommended, and *The Breast Cancer Notebook* described here can serve as a good model.

The protocol discussed in this book can be used in varying degrees for patients with different types of cancer, different stages of cancer, and other life-threatening illnesses. Some groups require more structure and education than others. *The Breast Cancer Notebook* and structured aspects of the protocol described here can help in developing such tools. Other groups are best facilitated with minimal structure, maximizing group interaction and allowing for spontaneous expression of concerns. The group facilitation style described in chapter 5 is optimal for enhancing this type of discussion. Whatever the therapists' style, the skills described in chapter 5 will maximize the benefit patients can derive from the group.

Various Clinical Settings

CANCER CENTERS

Those working in a major cancer center are fortunate in that they can conduct groups that are highly homogenous. It should also be possible to find therapists who can work in pairs and complement each other. Because National Cancer Institute Comprehensive Cancer Centers are required to have a strong psychosocial component, little justification is usually needed for conducting groups for cancer patients.

HOSPITALS

Therapists who work in large hospitals may need to compromise on homogeneity to some extent. They may need to decide whether to form groups on the basis of disease type or severity of disease. Yet an even more difficult issue is how to justify to hospital administration the value of such a group. Certainly competition in health markets will help administrators appreciate that conducting cancer groups presents their hospital in a friendlier light to patients, which can attract more patients to their site. This argument may not be as useful for managed care (especially health maintenance organizations), where attracting cancer patients (with their costly treatments) may be seen as a financial liability. However, it is useful for staff therapists to point out that

▪ it is more economical for therapists to see 10 patients once a week than to see individual patients 10 times a week.
▪ patients attending a regular group are less likely to make unnecessary medical appointments and more likely to make necessary medical appointments.

Furthermore, policies in large institutions are slow to change, so therapists who are tasked with conducting cancer groups usually have the backing of the entire institution for some time to come, which is important for recruitment. Although recruitment should be relatively easy in a large institution, in truth it can be surprisingly difficult. To improve recruitment, it may be necessary to give several in-service presentations to oncology, radiation oncology, and surgery department staffs. Nurses, as well as front desk staff, often refer more patients than the doctors themselves. Finally, it will probably be necessary to inform the patients themselves about the groups through posters and brochures in the waiting room. Ideally, it is useful to have a flier handed out to every newly diagnosed patient and to send a mailing from their physician at the 6-month postdiagnosis mark (close to end-of-treatment). Although the most convenient time for therapists to contact patients, and arguably the most important time for patients to be contacted, is immediately after diagnosis, this is also the least likely time for most patients to begin group therapy. Still, offering some initial support, with invitations for later follow-up, is a valuable service.

SMALL CLINICS AND PRIVATE PRACTICE

Therapists who work at small medical or psychological clinics or who wish to conduct groups on their own may wish to develop a psychooncology service both for their own patients and also for the community. The benefits of offering this service at a small clinic or on one's own is that therapists can develop the type of group they believe is most effective. The drawbacks, however, are centered mainly on finances. Advertising costs, therapists' salaries, workbook supplies, and so on must be reimbursed from patient fees. Therefore, groups will only continue as long as there are a sufficient number of paying patients.

Licensed mental health professionals can bill for group psychotherapy (Procedure Code 90853) and use the *Diagnostic and Statistical Manual of Mental Disorders* (4th ed.; American Psychiatric Association, 1994) or the *International Classification of Disease* (10th ed.; World Health Organization, 1996) diagnostic code 316.00 (Psychological Factors Affecting Physical Condition, specifically Distress Affecting Coping With Cancer), or one of the Adjustment Disorders (309), or even Pain Disorder with Both Medical and Psychological Factors (307.89). Even the most stringently managed care companies are likely to approve group therapy when there is a medical necessity. Managed care, however, may restrict the number of group therapy sessions they allow the patient to attend (typically 8), and it may be up to therapists to justify continued psychological treatment.

Whatever the setting, it is well worth the effort to coordinate group psychotherapy for cancer patients. Patients need it, and for therapists it is both economical and emotionally satisfying.

Conclusion

In this book, we have offered a specific model of group psychotherapy for women with breast cancer. We have described this model in such a way that therapists with lesser experience can follow it closely, whereas those who have been conducting these types of groups can take what they find useful and integrate it into their own style of therapy. We have made every effort to base the recommendations in this book on what has been demonstrated to be effective in the research literature and through extensive clinical experience, but we recognize that therapy is as much an art as a science. Each therapist has a unique sensitivity, personality, and experience and therefore must ultimately find his or her way in providing therapy to patients. We hope that this book has provided some support for that endeavor.

Although the focus of this book has been on treating breast cancer per se, we have found this approach to be effective in the treatment of a wide range of medical illnesses. For those who find the approach discussed here of value, extending these tools to other cancers and life-threatening illnesses should not be overly difficult.

Appendix

Structured Existential Exercises

Structured exercises beyond those used in the early sessions can be introduced to get the group to actively and authentically discuss serious concerns. Exercises may be helpful when it is necessary to accentuate an important point that the group appears to have difficulty grasping through normal facilitative intervention. Exercises can also be introduced when the group seems to be stagnating, does not respond to therapeutic prompts, or stays external, abstract, and intellectual despite therapists' best efforts to redirect to meaningful expression. Exercises, however, are no substitute for group discussion and interaction. Rather, they should only be used when such interaction is lacking and as a way to stimulate renewed discussion. As stated in chapters 4–6, these exercises should be used with caution and only as a last resort. If this occurs more than once or twice during the life of a particular group, close examination of the dynamics leading to this and consultation with other therapists may be warranted.

The following is a sampling of exercises that have been used extensively in groups for breast cancer patients. Based on "Existential Group Psychotherapy for Women With Advanced Breast Cancer and Other Life-Threatening Illnesses," by J. Spira, in *Group Psychotherapy for Medically Ill Patients* (165–224), edited by J. Spira, 1997b, New York: Guilford Press. Copyright 1997 by Guilford Press. Adapted with permission.

CHANGING SELF

Everyone has a self-image, although most people are unaware of it. Yet one's image of oneself can both spur one to excel or limit one's potential.

When struck with cancer, one may be reluctant to adapt to changing circumstances because one clings to a precancer view of oneself. If patients are having difficulty adjusting to current circumstances, this simple exercise can begin to reveal the tendency to form self-images that become fixed and the possibility of considering alternatives.

What goes into your self-image? (Factors may include positive or negative aspects of body image, personality characteristics, beliefs, things you do, people you know, and so on.)

1. Write down the 10 most important aspects of your self-image, those things without which you would not have been you.
2. Write down what your self-image was like when you were 20 years old.
3. Write down what your future self-image might be like 6 months before you die.
4. Is one more accurate? How does self-image affect what you do and how you do it?

PORTRAIT EXERCISE

The following exercise is helpful when group members have expressed (consciously or unconsciously) feeling trapped in their lives or life circumstances.

Draw two rectangles.

1. The left rectangle can be considered the portrait of you that has been drawn up to this point. Inside the frame write down aspects of yourself that comprise your self-image. These could be positive or negative personality characteristics, beliefs, things you do, people you know, how you look, and so on.
2. Outside the rectangle list those factors that have contributed to your current self-image. These can include genetics, early family environment, families' social-economic status, early schooling, later choice of relationships, and work.
3. Consider how much of your current self-image and activities have been chosen for you as opposed to chosen by you.
4. Now look at the blank portrait to the right. If you could draw your self-image in 1 year, the way you'd like it to be (given constraints out of one's control, such as genetics, illness, etc.), how would you choose this portrait to be? Inside, write down the characteristics you'd most respect in yourself. Outside, put the activities in which you'd most like to engage.

5. What is preventing you from becoming more like the rectangle on the right, and how can you move more toward that in your life?

BELIEFS EXERCISE

Most of us are unaware of fundamental beliefs that guide our actions and constrain our consideration of what is possible. When fundamental beliefs and attitudes are clearly limiting patients' lives, the following "beliefs" exercise is helpful.

There are many beliefs, attitudes, and characteristics we developed early in our lives that are still with us and influence the way we see the world and the decisions we make. For example, if one believes that others are fundamentally separate from us, and everyone has to fend for themselves and get what they can from others, then it will be natural to be suspicious of others and to remain vigilant, to become aggressive in protecting one's own interests, to be at a greater stage of physiological readiness, and to be especially competitive to secure one's position. If, on the other hand, one believes that one is incapable of achieving success, that the world is uncaring and unsupportive, and that the future holds no possibility of improvement, then one inevitably experiences depressive thoughts, flat emotions, low physiological arousal, and little motivation to work. Thus, our attitudes about ourselves and our world influence the way we act. Other beliefs include having to be "perfect," believing that one is not fundamentally a good person, having to take care of others before oneself, never showing emotions, and so on.

1. Write down a belief, characteristic, or attitude you have about yourself, others, or your world that may negatively affect your quality of life.
2. When was this belief formed? What were the circumstances at that time?
3. How did this belief serve you well at that time?
4. How does this belief still serve you well?
5. How does this belief limit you now?
6. What alternative belief, attitude, or characteristic would be beneficial to have in order to complement the old belief, so that you could use whichever is most useful in various situations?

ORPHEUS EXERCISE

A cancer patient, like anyone else, has difficulty letting go of views of oneself in order to adjust to changes in circumstances. However, cancer patients' "selves" are changing all the time. A woman's sense of femininity and sexuality must change when she has a mastectomy, hair loss, sudden menopause, vaginal dryness, and loss of libido and vitality. A sense of motherhood is threatened when she is too tired, in too much pain, or too busy with medical appointments to go to a child's school functions, cook meals, or help with homework. The following powerful exercise (inspired by one described by James Bugental, 1973/4) helps cancer patients accept and grieve their loss and at the same time consider what they might find at their core.

1. Write down the 10 most important aspects of your self-image, those things without which you would not have been you. (These can include positive or negative aspects of body image, personality characteristics, beliefs, things you do, people you know, and so on.)
2. Now rank order these aspects of yourself, with 10 being least central and 1 being most central to your self-image.
3. Next, take number 10 in your list, and cross it out. Take a minute to imagine what your life would be like without this aspect of yourself. When you can do that, do the same with number 9 and every other number until you finish with number 1. (When you finish, notice that some of the items might have been very difficult for you to cross off, whereas you may have been happy to remove others.)
4. Now, turn the page over. Write down the two or three most important characteristics you would like to have, if you could now re-create the type of self-image you would like, that would allow you to live as fully as possible in the future.

ONE YEAR TO LIVE

This exercise helps patients focus on their illness as an opportunity for growth.

If you had only one year to live:

1. What personality characteristics would you like to get rid of?
2. What activities would you want to cease doing?
3. What personality characteristics would you want to have in order to be able to live your life more fully and enjoyably?
4. What activities would you like to be engaged in that would give your life most meaning and value?
5. What is stopping you from making these changes now?
6. What can you do to overcome these barriers?

PRIORITIES EXERCISE

The following exercise encourages patients to use the crisis of the illness as an opportunity to reevaluate their priorities so that they can focus on what is most important in their lives.

Draw three columns on your page.

1. In column 1, list the 10 major activities you are engaged in during a typical week.
2. In column 2, prioritize these items, ordering them in terms of which activity you spend the most time with on top, and the items you spend the least time with on the bottom.
3. In column 3, reprioritize the items, but this time, list the activity that brings most meaning to you, those items that make life worth living, on top, and the items of lessening personal value toward the bottom. You may also wish to add new items to the list that you wish you could get to but don't usually have the time.
4. Draw lines between similar items in column 2 and 3. If you have large Xs, or if your lines go mostly straight across, what does this mean to you?
5. What can you do to spend more time engaged in those activities that make your life worth living? What do you have to reduce or eliminate in order to bring this more centrally into your life?

Meditation Exercises

The following is a more detailed description of Zen-based meditation adapted for a medically ill population. Several introductory exercises are presented which patients find relatively easy to learn, practice, and benefit from. (Note: These exercises are adapted from Spira, 1994.)

Basic Posture

1. Sitting on the edge of a chair, if possible, is best. If your back gets too fatigued, then sit at the very back of a firm chair, but role your back away from the back of the chair. If you have a back injury, and your back tends to go into spasms or have sharp or cutting pain, then rest against the back of the chair.
2. Have your feet flat on the floor, directly underneath your knees; separate your knees by a few inches.

3. Sit with your bones firmly pressing into the chair, not rolled forward or back.
4. Keep your chest up and chin in (with the back of your neck tall, toward the ceiling).
5. Place your right hand in your lap, palm up, just above the pubic bone (rested on the folds of your pants or dress); left hand is palm up and resting inside your right hand. The fingers overlap, the thumbs touch each other very gently, and also gently touch your navel. (If you become tense, you notice that you are pressing your hands or thumbs against each other or your navel; if you "space out," you notice that your thumbs come away from each other or your navel.)
6. With your eyes open, gaze downward on one area.
7. Keep your mouth closed and your teeth lightly touching, with your tongue up along the roof of your mouth and the tip of your tongue touching the teeth. You might also find it helpful to suck the air out of your mouth in order to create a slight suction.

General Instructions

No matter what the particular meditation exercise you are focusing on, whenever you become distracted (to an external or internal distraction), just let that go, and return your attention to the exercise. Rather than trying not to think of your distractions, instead just focus more fully on the exercise you are doing. If you find it difficult to concentrate, move to a more complex exercise (such as Tai Chi, sitting-moving meditation, or counting the breaths). Also, redouble your effort to focus as much as you can on the exercise as if your life depended on it. Have faith that this is the most important thing in the world at this very moment, and everything else depends on how well you can do this exercise. These exercises are not meant to put you to sleep—quite the opposite. The intention is to assist you in waking up fully, with effortless, calm, alertness, allowing you to be more fully present in this very moment.

SITTING-MOVING MEDITATION

Purpose

The more active and complex the exercise, the easier it is to focus on the moment. Thus, these sitting-moving exercises help you focus more fully in the moment, especially unifying mind and body (because attention must focus on body movements). These movements are also very healthy; moving your spine in a balanced way can reduce muscular-skeletal strain, massage the internal organs, and facilitate circulation of cerebral-spinal fluid throughout the central nervous system. However, the more complex and active the meditation, the easier it is to avoid habits and personality patterns. Thus, although this form of meditation can serve as a valuable first step in developing concentration and mind-body unity (when one is learning meditation or for the first few minutes of one's daily meditation routine), it is not the most powerful or valuable technique in the long run.

Methods

Sitting on the edge of your chair, with your feet solid on the floor underneath you, feel the breath. Follow your breath; don't force it. In fact, for an especially powerful experience, let the breath go a little bit more at the bottom of each exhalation. That is, whenever you exhale, at the bottom of the exhalation, let go of a little more air, and rest for a moment longer at the bottom of the breath (effortlessly, without forcing the breath out or holding it out) until the next breath automatically comes in.

1. As you inhale, arch forward; bring your spine forward, breath into the chest as it floats up, look up, and roll your tailbone back (forming a forward "C" in the spine).
2. As you exhale, relax back to the center; let your eyes rest to the center, your spine rest to the center, and your tailbone come back to the center.
3. As you inhale, arch backward; allow the breath to flow into your back as you arch your spine back, relax your chest down, and look downward to see the tail curling under.
4. As you exhale, relax back to the center; let your eyes rest to the center, your spine rest to the center, and your tailbone come back to the center.

   Repeat the movement for at least 12 inhalations and exhalations (keeping count during the movements). Follow the natural changes in the breath; don't force it.

Repeat the following exercise for at least 12 inhalations and exhalations (keeping count during the movements). Follow the natural changes in the breath; don't force it.

5. As you inhale, shift your weight to the left side, letting your ribs shift over to the left, and keeping your head and tail to the center (forming a sideways "C"). Turn your head and look at your right hip come up an inch off the chair.
6. As you exhale, relax back to the center.
7. As you inhale, shift your weight to the right side, letting your

ribs shift over to the right, and keeping your head and tail to the center (forming a sideways "C"). Turn your head and look at your left hip come up an inch off the chair.

8. As you exhale, relax back to the center.

Repeat the following exercise for at least 12 inhalations and exhalations (keeping count during the movements). Follow the natural changes in the breath; don't force it.

9. As you inhale, rotate to the left, lifting your pubic bone and rotating to the left, then lifting your chest and rotating to the left, then tucking in your chin and rotating to the left, and then finally turning your eyes all the way to the left to look at your left shoulder.

10. As you exhale, relax back to the center.

11. As you inhale, rotate to the right, lifting your pubic bone and rotating to the right, then lifting your chest and rotating to the right, then tucking in your chin and rotating to the right, and then finally turning your eyes all the way to the right to look at your right shoulder.

12. As you exhale, relax back to the center.

Results Over Time

You can do this as the first part of your daily meditation practice to help begin to unify your mind and body and bring yourself into the moment. Or you can do this as your only meditation practice, especially if you are just learning meditation or if you feel especially "noisy" and distracted that day. In this case, do four sets of the above exercise.

At first, it is natural to feel very calm and a general sense of well-being resulting from this meditation practice. If you began by feeling tired or drained, you may feel more calmly alert and ready for activity. If you began by feeling "keyed up" or agitated, you will no doubt feel calmer and more relaxed, perhaps even sleepy. At first, especially if you are ill, you may find it beneficial to lie down after doing this exercise, in order to "balance the system." Then, you should be able to approach the day feeling more calm, clear, comfortable, and alert (without agitation).

BREATH AWARENESS MEDITATION

Purpose

Not as active as the sitting-moving meditation (above), breath awareness meditation is one of the most traditional and commonly practiced meditation practices—and for good reason. This practice helps to increase mental alertness, physical and mental calm, awareness of one's habit thoughts, unconscious fears and desires, and control over previously uncontrollable impulses and habits. Moreover, in being able to become aware of the breath without pushing it or pulling it, we also can learn to become aware of other people and things without habitually and unnecessarily manipulating them in our minds. Thus, we can come to appreciate the world "as it is," without our constant manipulation of it as a result of our unconscious and habitual fears and desires.

Methods

A variety of breath awareness exercises can be practiced. These range from the more active and complex (and thus easier to begin with) to the simpler and therefore more powerful (in terms of the above benefits). Presented below is a simple yet powerful breath-oriented meditation.

1. Awareness of the breath at different parts of your body, for six breaths each.

- Touch with your fingers the area into which you breathe. When you inhale, breathe into one part of your body, touch that area with your finger tips, and release from that area. Begin with your nose for six breaths, and then move to your chest, belly, lower back, midback, and upper back, for six breaths each. Repeat this circle six times. Do not force the breath. Rather, just simply notice how the breath is occurring at that area.
- Notice major areas into which you breathe. When you inhale, breathe into and out of one part of your body, noticing how that area expands into and release from that area. Notice every subtle aspect of this; how the temperature and texture change from the inhalation to the exhalation, how the place that expands and releases feels, and so on. Begin with your nose for six breaths, and then move to your chest, belly, lower back, midback, and upper back, for six breaths each. Repeat this circle at least six times. Do not force the breath. Rather, just simply notice how the breath is occurring at that area.

2. Awareness of the breath flowing down the front and up the back. As above, notice the breath flowing into one area of your body, but now for only one breath at one area at a time. Become aware of the breath flowing into and out of your nose. For the next breath, drop your awareness down 2 inches to your upper throat, and so on down the front, under the pelvis, and up the back, over the head, one area for one breath. Make this circle at least six times.

3. Simple breath awareness. Sit still, with awareness of the breath expanding and releasing simultaneously into and out of every cell of the body, as if you are a balloon, expanding and releasing equally everywhere in all directions. As you sit, with eyes, ears, and all the senses open, notice that your front, sides, and back all expand and release together at the same time.

It may take all the attentional effort you can gather in order to stay fully absorbed in the breath. The more you pour yourself into the exhalation and drink in the inhalation with every ounce of effort you can muster, the sooner you can suspend any effort and simply allow the breath to breathe you. The more attentional effort you make, the less energy will be available for habit thinking. Alternate between this supreme effort and this supreme effortlessness as needed. This corresponds to the manifesting of the self and the release of the self. Eventually, your energy will be indistinct from the natural energy of the world.

Results

The more you can be present without reflection while sitting, the more fully you can engage in everything and anything you do. Initially, the more frequently you can recognize that you have begun reflecting during the sitting and bring yourself back to the present moment, the more control you will have over your mind and emotions.

Early in your practice, you may sense that there is signal (present moment) and noise (random thoughts) existing side by side during the meditation. The more effort you give to the moment at hand (the sensory light, sound, tactile sensations), the less energy there will be to maintain the activity of "noise," and it will soon disappear, leaving just the moment at hand. Be gentle, but persistent. Occasionally, intense pleasure or distress will arise. This might manifest as physical pain or agitation, pleasure or intense energy, visual images or memories, thoughts or sounds. Fears of safety or death may arise as you begin letting go of your image of yourself, others, and the world. You may be conscious of this, or it may manifest as increased dissociation into daydreams or focusing on pleasant memories or body feelings (covering up one's *angst*). Whatever arises, simply notice it, accept it fully as you inhale, release it fully as you exhale, and then turn to the sensations immediately in front of you and let yourself be absorbed in what you see, hear, and feel. Eventually, you will be able to sit and breathe with all the world flowing in and out—thus returning to the natural condition of existence and being able to act more fully from this fundamental place.

Results Over Time

Practicing these breath awareness methods on a twice-daily basis (morning and evening for at least 20 minutes each) results in improved

- awareness of your body;
- feelings of health and energy in body and mind;
- feelings of physical comfort and psychological well-being;
- awareness of previously unconscious habits, fears, and desires;
- control over your impulses, and the ability to make healthy choices; and
- mental clarity.

Self-Hypnosis Methods

Hypnosis is simply the volitional shifting of consciousness into a normal and natural recuperative and creative state that we typically enter into many times throughout the day. The exercises listed below permit individuals to enter into this state for a brief period to (a) relax, (b) consider difficult issues that might otherwise appear to be too overwhelming, and (c) consider creative solutions to one's problems.

There are three phases to therapeutic hypnosis: induction phase, utilization phase, and integration phase. The following exercises assist in induction. We then offer several examples of applications to use while in a light hypnotic state or for imagery during relaxation. As with any psychotherapeutic technique, anyone who wishes to use such methods must undergo sufficient training and have experience and supervision.

INDUCTION

Induction Into a Light Trance State

If this is the patient's first experience with hypnosis, explain hypnosis as a normal and natural recuperative state.

(read very slowly, breaking at each comma) Sitting comfortably in your chair, letting your body sink into the chair, and noticing your breath flow in and out. Notice your chest rising with the inhalation . . . With the next inhalation squeeze your hands, raise your shoulders, take a deep breath in, and hold it, and let your eyes look up toward the ceiling. As you continue to look up and hold your breath, let your eyelids slowly close. When your eyelids touch, JUST LET GO. (Release and lower your own voice.)

Let go of your eyes, breath, shoulders, and hands . . . And feel your mind and body relaxing. Let your mind relax so much it feels as if it can float, free and easy, safe and secure. Feel as if your mind is able to relax into your breath, and your breath can relax into your body And your body can relax into the chair. And the chair can sink into the floor. Allow the floor to support the chair, and the chair to support your body. And your body to comfort and relax you as the breath effortlessly massages you, and lets your mind float effortlessly and easily.

For initial assessment:

And as your body continues to comfort and relax you, keep you safe and secure, imagine a scene off in the distance,

- and in that scene imagine a setting where you are able to think and act with optimal health and clarity, where you feel and look and sound calm and happy and competent, and where you are able to be the way you'd like to be. You may have been this way before, or you may be able to imagine how nice it would be in the future to be this way. (Pause for 5 breaths.)

Then, knowing that you can return to this place whenever you need to or want to

- bring this feeling back with you, as you
- notice your inhalation raising your chest up (your voice raises up and becomes a little louder and faster)
- and with the next breath or the one after, allow your eyes and eyelids to float up—up with the next inhalation, then refocusing on the room, feeling good clear, calm, energetic to help you through the rest of the day.

(Debrief)

Induction Into a Deeper Trance State

Begin as above, but instead of imagining a scene off in the distance, tell patients the following:

As you continue to let the chair soothe and support your body, and as you continue to let your body soothe and support your mind:

Imagine that you are in a very wonderful and nurturing environment. You might be inside or outside, whatever comes to you most easily and effortlessly. You can make this place as perfect as need be. After all, this is the realm of imagination, where everything can be just perfect. Enjoy being in this place. Notice what's around you, and how nice it is to be here.

Now look off into the distance, and notice that about 30 steps away is an even more wonderful place, a special healing place, where you can completely relax your mind and body, and allow that place to nurture you and refresh you and heal any physical or mental distress. This is a place you can trust completely, because it is your own unconscious mind. Your unconscious contains all the resources you need to help you, keep you safe and protect you. And this is a very creative place as well, where once you relax your conscious mind, your unconscious can provide you with solutions to your problems.

▌ In a moment I will ask you to begin walking toward this wonderful healing place. Next time I say the word "NOW," you can take a step toward it. And the breath will help you move there effortlessly and easily. Since it is now 30 steps away, with each step, you can count another number, backward from 30.

▌ Ready . . . with the next exhalation, you can take step number "29." NOW . . . . .

▌ With each breath, with each step, as you count backward, you will find yourself getting closer to that wonderful and special healing place. . . . And as you get closer, you will begin to feel the gentle power of this place touching you, and helping you float more effortlessly toward it.

▌ It's nice to be able to JUST LET GO AND RELAX, trusting that the breath and your unconscious mind is helping you to reach this wonderful place, this effortless state. And as you continue to walk along, with each breath, counting one number down with each step . . .

▌ you can JUST LET GO of whatever you no longer need to carry along with you . . . you can simply set it aside along the path (you can pick it up later if you like, on your way back, or you can let it stay, whatever is best for you).

▌ and you can FIND WHATEVER YOU NEED along the way to help you more easily reach this wonderful healing and creative place. You might encounter a person, or an animal, or some special object to help you. Or you might simply notice some color or sound or feeling that is helping you along.

▌ and you don't even have to listen consciously to my voice, because your unconscious can understand what I'm saying, and will take what's useful and let go of what is not useful, to help you. And my voice will go with you into this wonderful place.

▌ and as you approach the final few steps, you can finally let go of any unnecessary tension or effort or consciousness, as your unconscious accepts you fully into this wonderful healing and creative place. And you can let go NOW.

UTILIZATION

Various imagery techniques are described in the next section.

It's nice to be able to trust your unconscious to help you and heal you.

And it's nice to know that you can return here whenever you need to or want to, simply by taking a deep breath in, Squeezing your hands and shoulders and looking up, Slowly closing your eyelids and then, letting go and relaxing completely.

When you feel relaxed, comfortable, calm, clear, and able to let your body soothe and comfort you, then imagine this wonderful place, off in the distance, and then take one step with each exhalation, as you count backward from 30, until you get there.

You can stay there as long as you like, trusting that your body and mind will help you to solve your problem.

But for now,

Knowing that you can return here whenever you like

You can begin to come back up this path, floating up five steps with each inhalation

Bringing back this good feeling and calm, clear energy with you,

And bringing back whatever else your unconscious has provided for you,

As you TAKE DEEPER INHALATIONS, coming up toward this room, bringing all the benefit of the hypnosis with you.

And in these last few inhales, you can BREATHE EVEN DEEPER INTO YOUR CHEST, noticing your chest rise up with the inhale,

And in the next inhale or the one after, allow your eyes and eyelids to RISE UP, up to the ceiling, and then refocus on the room feeling clear and alert with good calm energy.

(Debrief)

SELF-HYPNOSIS AND IMAGERY TECHNIQUES

Whether therapists wish to induce a hypnotic state with the above methods or simply use a relaxation technique to help patients to achieve a state of comfort, the following are helpful exercises for summarizing the theme of the group, helping patients consider them more deeply and possibly in ways they have not previously considered.

The following are five basic aspects of the imagery–hypnosis session.

Use of Imagery Techniques

1. Help patients achieve a relaxed state.
2. Ask patients to imagine a scene off in the distance that contains some problem scenario. Ask them about the visual, auditory, and kinesthetic sensations they imagine in that scene.
3. Ask patients to imagine a new optimal way of handling that situation. Ask them about the visual, auditory, and kinesthetic sensations they imagine in that scene.
4. Ask patients what resources they need to be able to handle that situation in a more optimal way in the future.
5. Ask patients to imagine that, next time that situation occurs, they can begin handling the situation in a more optimal way.

Typical scenarios that might be used to summarize what occurred in the group session include the following:

Problem State:	Optimal State:
Habitual or negative reaction to a stressful situation	Optimal reaction to stressful situation
Afraid to acknowledge feelings (to self or others)	Comfortable expressing feelings (to self or others)
Out of control (or too much control)	Controlling what one can, letting go of what one cannot
Afraid to address an issue (insufficient resources)	Willing to address an issue (sufficient resources)
Feeling helpless	Feeling confident
Hopeless for ever living as one did	Hopeful for finding something of value in one's life
Isolated	Connected to someone, somewhere
Unable to say "no"	Able to set clear limits
Worrying or anxious	Calm, focused, in the moment
Unable to feel joy or happiness	Able to laugh and enjoy oneself

It is also possible to contrast two situations, both of which merit consideration:

Grieving the death of a friend (What that friend gave you)	Imagine saying goodbye (What did you give that friend)
What you have lost	What you have found

PAIN MANAGEMENT EXERCISES

Pain as an Experience

Pain is more than just the pain nerves firing. Our experience of pain involves physical, psychological, and social aspects as well. Although we sometimes can do little to change the nerve firing, we can vary our reaction to the pain, and thus change our experience of the pain. And often this in turn can influence the nerves themselves

The three pain management exercises that follow can be very helpful to reduce one's experience of pain, and if practiced regularly, can produce long-term benefits.

Method 1: Where Is the Pain?

This is useful for persons with low levels of pain who might have a concrete cognitive style.

Preliminary Considerations:

Acknowledge pain and worry, offer sympathy.

Recognize the patient's relative cognitive inflexibility.

Appreciate that the pain can seem overwhelming; the patient tends to focus on only pain (my life is pain).

Describe what you are doing, and why (pain is an experience, not just a nerve firing; often we increase the sensation and suffering of the pain by our reaction to the pain). This exercise will help reduce the reaction to the pain, and therefore help you control the pain.

1. *Induce a state of relaxation*
2. Go to the center of the pain (e.g., 5th lumbar vertebrae).
   (a) Describe it in as much detail as possible (first let them try; then offer alternatives):
   - *intensity:* Rate the intensity of the pain from 1 to 10.
   - *quality:* Is the pain sharp, dull, aching, cutting, throbbing, burning, stinging, etc.?
   - *frequency:* Is it continuous, coming and going, when resting, when moving, etc.?
   - *extent:* How far does it spread (where is it, where is it not)?
   (b) Go 1 inch out from the center of the pain.
   - Rate its intensity now.
   - Describe the quality and frequency now (same or different?).
   (c) Continue to go 1 inch out, as in (b), until there is no pain at that location.
3. Now describe what you feel at this more comfortable area.
   (a) Describe it in as much detail as possible (first let them try; then offer alternatives)
   - *quality:* What is the temperature (warm) or texture (soft);

is it stationary or moving (fluid); what is the energy (calm)?

- ▪ *extent:* Does this exist any where else in your body?
- ▪ *intensity:* On a scale of 1 to 10 of comfort, how strong is this feeling?

(b) Go 1 inch further in toward the center of that other feeling.
  - ▪ Do you feel any of that good feeling now?
  - ▪ Rate it on a scale of 1 to 10.

(c) Continue to go 1 inch in, as in (b), until there is still some good feeling there, even in the center (or around the center). Note that both sensations are there, but you can focus on the good sensation as much as the bad, or more.

The pain has been grabbing your attention. With practice, however, you can regain control over your attention.

Method 2: Merge Metaphors

Use this method for persons with moderate levels of pain who have a somewhat flexible cognitive style.

Preliminary Considerations:

1. Establish rapport on pain and distress it causes.
2. Ask the patient: "What is the pain like?"
3. Get a sense of how they represent the pain (visual–kinesthetic–auditory); use an optimal representational system.
4. Do they presently feel any comfort anywhere in their body? (If not: What is enjoyable to them? Can they recall feeling comfortable anywhere in their body?)

Attempt first to discover this resource currently in their body, and if that is too difficult then in the past in memory, and if need be in the future in imagination.

Merge Metaphor Technique:

Negative Metaphor:

1. *Induct into light trance:*
2. If the pain was a (color/sound/texture/or animal [c/s/t/a]; select according to their representational system) what (c/s/t/a) would it be? (Let them try first, and then offer examples if needed.)
3. Rate (c/s/t/a) on scale from 1 to 10. (From now on, only mention metaphor.)
4. Increase the intensity of the c/s/t/a one point (pause for 2 seconds, or ask the patient to raise a finger); then decrease several

points, allowing the c/s/t/a to fade/reduce/soften/become gentler (color on a screen; texture in an object; sound on a tape deck; animal in a cage).

5. *Repeat 4, once again with the therapist's lead, and then ask the patient to continue on her own a few times, until the c/s/t/a no longer further fades (or reduces, softens, or becomes gentler).*

Positive Metaphor:

1. Now focus on a comfortable area in your body (or mind, if necessary).
2. If the comfort was a c/s/t/a(same representational system), what c/s/t/a would it be? (Let them try first, and then offer examples, if needed.)
3. Rate c/s/t/a on scale from 1 to 10. (From now on, only mention metaphor.)
4. Allow the c/s/t/a to grow and begin to move toward the other one. Notice how it soothes you as it spreads throughout your body, coming to meet the other c/s/t/a.

Merge Metaphor:

Build tension: "In a moment, these two c/s/t/a will merge; I don't know how they will merge; and you don't either, consciously; but the unconscious will find a magical/creative way for this to occur."

1. Now allow the positive c/s/t/a's to come close to the other c/s/t/a. Let it encircle it. Then let them merge (pause for 30 seconds). Colors, textures, and animals can blend; sounds can be on two tape decks and blend in a room.
2. How has the c/s/t/a changed?
3. Now rate the merged c/s/t/a on a scale from 1 to 10.

Future Integration: Review the exercise. Then say: "It's nice to know that any time in the future you begin focusing on this negative c/s/t/a; you can reduce it and then allow the positive c/s/t/a to come to your assistance simply by doing this exercise."

Method 3: Distancing the Pain

This is useful for persons who have a great deal of cognitive flexibility and who can become easily absorbed in imagery.

Preliminaries:

Because these patients are very suggestible, (a) establish slight rapport on their concern, (b) don't dwell on the negative or go into too much detail or submodalities (visual, auditory, kinesthetic features of their pain representation), and (c) pace the potential success of using hypnosis for them; be confident and positive.

Get information: Ask them what a very pleasant and comforting place or activity is for them.

First, if possible, give them a good, deep trance or relaxation experience, free of pain and worry, and then, afterward, teach them a lighter trance self-hypnosis exercise that they can use on their own.

Induct into Moderate Trance or Deep State of Relaxation

Acknowledge pain and other distractions but state that they are "out there in the distance," whereas they are able to do this exercise at the center of their mind.

Instruct the patients to go to that comfortable place and activity we talked about before. (Note: In order to facilitate fuller absorption, don't suggest "*as if*" they were at that place, simply instruct them to "go there" directly.)

> Ask about the visual and auditory images they have; also inquire about the comfortable kinesthetic experiences, but keep these to a minimum since we want to distance them from the pain feeling and cognitive representation of pain. Ask them to describe the scene.

Discuss pain metaphorically: Ask them, "do you notice any discomfort?"

> If they respond, "no or not much," stay with the comfort, put a comfort screen around you that blocks the discomfort, even though you may notice that it is there, off in the distance.

> If they respond, "yes," ask them what the discomfort would be if it was part of the scenery. Work it into the scene in a distanced manner. (From then on, discuss only the metaphor, not the pain.)

> For example:

> ▪ if they are at the beach, and they experience the pain as waves crashing; state that the waves can be seen crashing over the bow of a boat, off in the distance, disturbing it for a moment, but then the boat can settle back down again.
> ▪ if they are in the forest, a loud crow can squawk occasionally, off in the distance, but then that will pass, or the crow will fly off a little further, so that the sound is further away, and they can notice the other pleasant sounds closer to them.

The therapist should continue as follows:

> ▪ Build the intensity of the submodalities (brighter, louder, closer vs. dimmer, quieter, further away).

▪ Alternate between acknowledging the intensity of distress out there in the distance (e.g., waves rising and sinking) and leading to comfort here at the center (beach).

▪ When pain intensifies, have them intensify the metaphor off in the distance. Then have them let that intensity subside and refocus back here, where they can focus on comfortable visual and auditory (and possibly kinesthetic) sensations.

There are many pain management techniques that are useful for cancer patients, including cognitive therapy, biofeedback, and even exercise. Yet self-hypnosis exercises discussed above work well in the type of group psychotherapy presented in this book, and at least one of these exercises should be useful to the majority of women in the group.

Therapist Forms

THERAPIST SELF-EVALUATION FORM

Although developed for evaluation of therapists in a multicenter research trial to determine whether therapists can effectively learn group therapy methods such as those described in this book, the following may be useful for review of how well one uses the basic skills emphasized here. (This form is based in part on Spira, 1991, and Spiegel & Spira, 1991, and was developed by James L. Spira for use by Spiegel, Morrow, & Clausen, 1999.)

_____ Absent _____ Adequate _____ Effective _____ Highly effective

_____ No opportunity to evaluate

Topics:

_____ helps initiate topics, when the group lacks relevant discussion

_____ keeps group on target, when needed

_____ introduces topics that have not been addressed, but which are of interest to the group, when needed

_____ integrates structured exercises seamlessly (in a way that seems natural to the group), when needed

Skills of rapport:

_____ non-verbally connected with group or particular patient engaged with (facial expressions, attentiveness, timing, etc.)

_____ verbally connected with group and particular patient engaged with (demonstrates understanding through paraphrases and summaries)

_____ follows group motivation (content and feeling that is appropriate for the meeting)

Leading skills:

_____ does not appear overly directive, but instead appears to allow exploration (Offers rapport before or in combination with leading; does not give information until others have an opportunity to come up with information, whenever appropriate)

_____ helps direct from external/general to personal/specific

_____ helps offer opportunity for expression of feelings

_____ helps offer opportunity for expression of thoughts

_____ elicits exploration of active coping solutions

_____ encourages interaction among group members

_____ encourages adaptation to current situation, and living more fully in the moment

Group cohesion, facilitates group cohesion through:

_____ helps members to support each other

_____ helps diffuse negative interpersonal feelings in group

_____ handles "problem" patients who dominate group

_____ handles "quiet" patients who have trouble participating in group

Group process:

_____ reflection about where group is heading, momentarily and over time

_____ handles negative emotions

_____ handles group confrontation of therapists or group in general

Other therapeutic skills:

THERAPIST CHECKLIST

Debriefing Following Each Group Meeting: Debriefing is an essential part of the group process.

After each group, co-therapists should take time to review factors related to the group.

Topics discussed in the group (lack of control, changes in self-image, etc.): (see topics discussed in chapter 5)

▪ Topics that should continue or related topics for next session:

Quality of group discussion (degree of affect, tendency to seek information, etc.): (See Tables 5.1 and 5.2)

▪ each group member's participation (concerns and quality of expression)
▪ member-related process considerations to keep in mind for future sessions

Debriefing among co-therapists should also consider the interaction between each therapist and the group, as well as between the co-therapists:

▪ How each therapist felt about the group as a whole (e.g., *Was the group dealing with critical issues, avoiding feelings, passive, etc.*)
▪ How each therapist felt about their activity in the group, as a whole (e.g., *I seemed to be a little too active this session, trying to help too much.* Or *I need to try to be less defensive with Joanne. I feel like she challenges me.*)
▪ Each therapist's emotional experience (e.g., *I got so sad when Maureen was talking about her daughter.*)
▪ How each therapist felt in their relationship to the other co-therapist (e.g., *I was annoyed with you because I felt like you cut Maureen off too soon.* Or *I felt that I jumped in too quickly to "help" you with Jean.*)

References

Adler, A., & Brett, C. (1998). *Social interest: Adler's key to the meaning of life*. Oxford, UK: OneWorld.

Ali, N. S., & Khalil, H. Z. (1989). Effect of pscyhoeducational intervention on anxiety among Egyptian bladder cancer patients. *Cancer Nursing, 12*, 236–242.

American Psychiatric Association. (1994). *Diagnostic and statistical manual of mental disorders* (4th ed.). Washington, DC: Author.

Andersen, B. L., Anderson, B., & deProsse, C. (1989). Controlled prospective longitudinal study of women with cancer: II. Psychological outcomes. *Journal of Consulting and Clinical Psychology, 57*, 692–697.

Andersen, B. L., Kiecolt-Glaser, J. K., & Glaser, R. (1994). A biobehavioral model of cancer stress and disease course. *American Psychologist, 49*, 389–404.

Antoni, M. (1997). Cognitive behavioral intervention for persons with HIV. In J. Spira (Ed.), *Group psychotherapy for medically ill patients* (pp. 55–91). New York: Guilford Press.

Ayres, A., Hoon, P. W., Franzoni, J. B., Matheny, K. B., Cotanch, P. H., & Takayanagi, S. (1994). Influence of mood and adjustment to cancer on compliance with chemotherapy among breast cancer patients. *Journal of Psychosomatic Research, 38*, 393–402.

Bandura, A., Blahard, E. B., & Ritter, B. (1969). Relative efficacy of desensitization and modeling approaches for inducing behavioral, affective, and attitudinal changes. *Journal of Personality and Social Psychology, 13*, 173–199.

Baum, A., & Anderson, B. (2001). *Psychosocial interventions for cancer*. Washington, DC: American Psychological Association.

Beck, A. T., Rush, A. J., Shaw, B. F., & Emery, G. (1979). *Cognitive therapy of depression*. New York: Guilford Press.

Ben-Eliyahu, S., Yirmiya, R., Liebeskind, J. C., Taylor, A. N., & Gale, R. P. (1991). Stress increases metastatic spread of a mammary tumor in rats: Evidence for mediation by the immune system. *Brain, Behavior, and Immunity, 5*, 193–205.

Benzera, E. E. (1990). Psychodynamic group therapy: A multiple treatment approach for private practice. *Psychiatric Annals, 20*, 375–378.

Binswanger, L. (1958). The existential analysis school of thought. In R. May, E. Angell, & H. Ellenberger (Eds.), *Existence* (pp. 48–192). New York: Simon & Schuster. (Original work published 1946)

Bugental, J. (1973/4). Confronting the existential meaning of "my death" through group exercises. *Interpersonal Development, 4,* 148–163.

Bugental, J. (1978). *Psychotherapy and process: The fundamentals of an existential-humanistic approach.* New York: Random House.

Cain, E. N., Kohorn, E. I., Quinlan, D. M., Latimer, K., & Schwartz, P. E. (1986). Psychosocial benefits of a cancer support group. *Cancer, 57,* 183–189.

Carkhuff, R. R. (2000). *The art of helping* (8th ed.). Amherst, MA: Human Resource Development Press.

Cassileth, B. R., Zupkis, R. V., Sutton-Smith, K., & March, V. (1980). Informed consent—Why are its goals imperfectly realized? *New England Journal of Medicine, 302,* 896–900.

Cella, D. F., & Tross, S. (1986). Psychological adjustment to survival from Hodgkin's disease. *Journal of Consulting and Clinical Psychology, 54,* 616–622.

Classen, C., Butler, L. D., Koopman, C., Miller, E., DiMiceli, S., Giese-Davis, J., et al. (2001). Supportive–expressive group therapy and distress in patients with metastatic breast cancer: A randomized clinical intervention trial. *Archives of General Psychiatry, 58*(5), 494–501.

Cordova, M. J., Andrykowski, M. A., Kenady, D. E., McGrath, P. C., Sloan, D. A., & Redd, W. H. (1995). Frequency and correlates of posttraumatic-stress-disorder-like symptoms after treatment for breast cancer. *Journal of Consulting and Clinical Psychology, 63,* 981–986.

Corey, G. (2000). *Theory and practice of group counseling* (5th ed.). Belmont, CA: Wadsworth.

Craig, T. J., & Abeloff, M. D. (1974). Symptomatology among hospitalized cancer patients. *American Journal of Psychiatry, 131,* 1323–1327.

Cunningham, A. J. (1989). A randomized trial of group psychoeducational therapy for cancer patients. *Patient Education and Counseling, 14,* 101–114.

Cunningham, A. J., Edmonds, C. V., Jenkins, G. P., Pollack, H., Lockwood, G. A., & Warr, D. (1998). A randomized controlled trial of the effects of group psychological therapy on survival in women with metastatic breast cancer. *Psychooncology, 7,* 508–517.

Derogatis, L. R., Abeloff, M. D., & Melisaratos, N. (1979). Psychological coping mechanisms and survival time in metastatic breast cancer. *Journal of the American Medical Association, 242,* 1504–1508.

Devine, E. C., & Westlake, S. K. (1995). The effects of psychoeducational care provided to adults with cancer: Meta-analysis of 116 studies. *Oncology Nursing Forum, 22,* 1369–1381.

Dunkel-Schetter, C., Feinstein, L. G., & Taylor, S. E. (1992). Patterns of coping with cancer. *Health Psychology, 11,* 79–87.

Edelman, S., Bell, D. R., & Kidman, A. D. (1999). A group cognitive behaviour therapy programme with metastatic breast cancer patients. *Psychooncology, 8,* 295–305.

Edmonds, C. V., Lockwood, G. A., & Cunningham, A. J. (1999). Psychological response to long-term group therapy: A randomized trial with metastatic breast cancer patients. *Psychooncology, 8,* 74–91.

Egan, G. (1973). *Face to face: The small-group experience and interpersonal growth.* London: Wadsworth.

Ellis, A. (1962). *Reason and emotion in psychotherapy.* New York: Lyle Stuart and Citadel Press.

Evans, R. L., & Connis, R. T. (1995). Comparison of brief group therapies for depressed cancer patients receiving radiation treatment. *Public Health Report, 110,* 306–311.

Fawzy, F. I., Cousins, N., Fawzy, N. W., Kemeny, M. E., Elashoff, R., & Morton, D. (1990). A structured psychiatric intervention for cancer patients: 1. Changes over time in methods of coping and affective disturbance. *Archives of General Psychiatry, 47,* 720–725.

Fawzy, F. I., Fawzy, N. W., Hyun, S. C., Elashoff, R., Guthrie, D., Fahey, J. L., et al. (1993). Malignant melanoma: Effects of an early structured psychiatric intervention, coping, and affective state on recurrence and survival 6 years later. *Archives of General Psychiatry, 50,* 681–689.

Fawzy, F. I., Fawzy, N. W., Hyun, C., & Wheeler, J. (1997). Brief coping-oriented therapy for patients with malignant melanoma. In J. Spira (Ed.), *Group psychotherapy for medically ill patients* (pp. 133–164). New York: Guilford Press.

Fawzy, F. I., Kemeny, M. E., Fawzy, N. W., Elashoff, R., Morton, D., Cousins, N., et al. (1990). A structured psychiatric intervention for cancer patients: II. Changes over time in immunological measures. *Archives of General Psychiatry, 47,* 729–735.

Forester, B., Kornfeld, D. S., Fleiss, J. L., & Thompson, S. (1993). Group psychotherapy during radiotherapy: Effects on emotional and physical distress. *American Journal of Psychiatry, 150,* 1700–1706.

Fox, B. H. (1998). A hypothesis about Spiegel et al.'s 1989 paper on psychosocial intervention and breast cancer survival. *Psychooncology, 7,* 361–370.

Gellert, G. A., Maxwell, R. M., & Siegel, B. S. (1993). Survival of breast cancer patients receiving adjunctive psychosocial support therapy: A 10-year follow-up study. *Journal of Clinical Oncology, 11,* 66–69.

Gendlin, E. (1979). Experiential psychotherapy. In R. Corsini (Ed.), *Current psychotherapies* (2nd ed., pp. 340–373). Itasca, IL: Peacock.

Glaser, B. G., & Strauss, A. L. (1967). *The discovery of grounded theory: Strategies for qualitative research.* New York: Adeline.

Glasser, W. (1965). *Reality therapy.* New York: Harper & Row.

Goodwin, P. J., Leszcz, M., Ennis, M., Koopmans, J., Vincent, L., Guther, H., et al. (2001). The effect of group psychosocial support on survival in metastatic breast cancer. *New England Journal of Medicine, 345,* 1719–1726.

Grunberg, N. E., & Baum, A. (1985). Biological commonalities of stress and substance abuse. In S. Shiffman & T. A. Wills (Eds.), *Coping and substance use* (pp. 25–62). San Diego, CA: Academic Press.

Haber, S. (Ed.). (1995). *Breast cancer: A psychological treatment manual.* New York: Springer.

Heidegger, M. (1962). Being and time (Macquarie & Robinson, Trans.). New York: Harper & Row. (Original work published in 1927)

Heinreich, R., & Schag, C. (1985). Stress and activity management: Group treatment for cancer patients and spouses. *Journal of Counseling and Clinical Psychology, 33,* 439–446.

Helgeson, V. S., Cohen, S., Schulz, R., & Yasko, J. (1999). Education and peer discussion group interventions and adjustment to breast cancer. *Archives of General Psychiatry, 56,* 340–347.

Helgeson, V. S., Cohen, S., Schulz, R., & Yasko, J. (2000). Group support interventions for women with breast cancer: Who benefits from what? *Health Psychology, 19,* 107–114.

Herberman, R. B. (1991). Principles of tumor immunology. In A. I. Holleb, D. J. Fink, & G. P. Murphy (Eds.), *Textbook of clinical oncology* (pp. 69–79). Atlanta, GA: American Cancer Society.

Holland, J. (1998). *Psychooncology.* New York: Oxford University Press.

Holland, J. (2001, December 17). Quoted in the *New York Times,* Section A, Page 36, Column 1.

Jamison, R. N., Burish, T. G., & Wallston, K. A. (1987). Psychogenic factors in predicting survival of breast cancer patients. *Journal of Clinical Oncology, 5,* 768–772.

Jaspers, K. (1994). *Philosophy of Existence.* Translated by R. F. Grabau. University of Pennsylvania Press.

Johnson, J. (1982). The effects of a patient education course on persons with a chronic illness. *Cancer Nursing, 117,* 117–123.

Kierkegaard, S. (1944). Either/Or. In R. Bretall (Ed.), A Kierkegaard Anthology (Swanson & Swanson, Trans.). Princeton, NJ: Princeton University Press.

Klerman, J. L., Weissman, M. M., Rounsavill, B. J., & Chevron, E. S. (1984). *Interpersonal psychotherapy of depression* (pp. 87–152). New York: Basic Books.

Levy, S. M., Lee, J., Bagley, C., & Lippman, M. (1988). Survival hazards analysis in first recurrent breast cancer patients: Seven-year follow-up. *Psychosomatic Medicine, 50,* 520–528.

Maslow, A. (1968). *Toward a psychology of*

being (2nd ed.). Princeton, NJ: Insight Books.

Massion, A. O., Teas, J., Hebert, J. R., Wertheimer, M. D., & Kabat-Zinn, J. (1995). Meditation, melatonin and breast/prostate cancer: Hypothesis and preliminary data. *Medical Hypotheses, 44*(1), 39–46.

Meyer, J., & Mark, M. M. (1995). Effects of psychosocial interventions with adult cancer patients: A meta-analysis of randomized experiments. *Health Psychology, 14*, 101–108.

Mitchell, J., & Everly, G. (1993). *Critical incident stress debriefing: CISD.* Ellicott City, MD: Chevron.

Nietzsche, F. (1967). *The will to power* (W. Kaufmann, Trans.). New York: Vintage. (Original notes completed 1888)

Perls, F. S. (1969). *Gestalt therapy verbatim.* Moab, UT: Real People Press.

Piaget, J. (1990). The equilibration of cognitive structures: The central problem of intellectual development. (Terence A. Brown, Translator & Kishore J. Thampy, Translator). Chicago: University of Chicago Press.

Plumb, M. M., & Holland, J. (1977). Comparative studies of psychological function in patients with advanced cancer: 1. Self-reported depressive symptoms. *Psychosomatic Medicine, 39*, 264–276.

Reed, G. M., & Stanton, A. L. (2002). *A model of brief group psychotherapy for symptomatic HIV-positive individuals.*

Richardson, J. L., Marks, G., Johnson, C. A., Graham, J. W., Chan, K. K., Selser, J. N., et al. (1987). Path model of multidimensional compliance with cancer therapy. *Health Psychology, 6*, 183–207.

Richardson, J. L., Marks, G., & Levine, A. (1988). The influence of symptoms of disease and side effects of treatment on compliance with cancer therapy. *Journal of Clinical Oncology, 6*, 1746–1752.

Rogentine, G. N., Jr., van Kammen, D. P., Fox, B. H., Docherty, J. P., Rosenblatt, J. E., Boyd, S. C., et al. (1979). Psychological factors in the prognosis of malignant melanoma: A prospective study. *Psychosomatic Medicine, 41*, 647–655.

Rogers, C. (1961). *On becoming a person: A therapist's view of psychotherapy.* New York: Houghton Mifflin.

Roter, D. L., Hall, J. A., Kern, D. E., Barker, L. R., Cole, K. A., & Roca, R. P. (1995). Improving physicians' interviewing skills and reducing patients' emotional distress. *Archives of Internal Medicine, 155*, 1877–1884.

Seligman, M. (1998). *Learned optimism.* New York: Simon & Schuster.

Siegel, B. (1988). *Love, medicine, and miracles: Self-healing from a surgeon's experience with exceptional patients.* New York: Harper Trade.

Siegel, B., Spira, J., & Ulmer, D. (1992, December). *The effects of group therapy on medically ill patients.* Panel discussion presented at the Fourth Annual Mind, Body, and Immunity Conference, Hilton Head, SC.

Simonton, C. O. (1995). *Cancer recovery and recurrence prevention.* Carlsbad, CA: Hay House, Inc.

Speice, J., Harkness, H., Laneri, R., Frankel, D., Roter, A., Kornblith, T., et al. (2000). Involving family members in cancer care: Focus group considerations of patients and oncological providers. *Journal of Psychooncology*, 101–112.

Spiegel, D., Bloom, J. R., Kraemer, H. C., & Gottheil, E. (1989). Effect of psychosocial treatment on survival of patients with metastatic breast cancer. *Lancet, 2*, 888–891.

Spiegel, D., Bloom, J. R., & Yalom, I. D. (1981). Group support for metastatic cancer patients: A randomized prospective outcome study. *Archives of General Psychiatry, 38*, 527–533.

Spiegel, D., & Glafkides, M. (1983). Effects of group confrontation with death and dying. *International Journal of Group Psychotherapy, 33*, 433–447.

Spiegel, D., Morrow, G. R., Classen, C., Raubertas, R., Stott, P. B., Mudaliar, N., et al. (1999). Group psychotherapy for recently diagnosed breast cancer patients: A multicenter feasibility study. *Psychooncology, 8*, 482–493.

Spiegel, D., & Spira, J. (1991). *Supportive-expressive group therapy: A treatment manual of psychosocial intervention for women with recurrent breast cancer.* Stanford, CA: Stanford University School of Medicine.

Spira, J. (1991). *Educational therapy: Existential, educational, and counseling approaches to behavioral medicine intervention.* Unpublished doctoral dissertation, University of California, Berkeley.

Spira, J. (1994). *Tai Chi Chuan and Zen meditation for the medically ill: Videotape and manual.* (Available from The Institute for Health Psychology, San Diego, CA.)

Spira, J. (1997a). Existential group psychotherapy for women with advanced breast cancer and other life-threatening illnesses. In J. Spira (Ed.), *Group psychotherapy for medically ill patients* (pp. 165–224). New York: Guilford Press.

Spira, J. (1997b). *Group psychotherapy for medically ill patients.* New York: Guilford Press.

Spira, J. (1997c). Understanding and developing psychotherapy groups for medically ill patients. In J. Spira (Ed), *Group psychotherapy for medically ill patients* (pp. 3–54). New York: Guilford Press.

Spira, J. (1998). Group psychotherapy for persons with cancer. In J. Holland (Ed.), *Psychooncology* (pp. 701–716). New York: Oxford University Press.

Spira, J. (2000). Existential psychotherapy in palliative care. Psychotherapy in palliative care. In H. M. Chochinov & W. Breitbart (Eds.), *Handbook of psychiatry in palliative medicine* (pp. 197–214). New York: Oxford University Press.

Spira, J., & Reed, G. (1996). Group psychotherapy for persons with first occurrence breast cancer. *A treatment manual for demonstration project by Blue Cross of Massachusetts, Inc. and the American Psychological Association Office of the Practice Directorate.* Unpublished manuscript.

Spira, J., & Spiegel, D. (1992). Hypnosis and related techniques in pain management for the terminally ill. *Hospice Journal,* 8(1/2), 89–120.

Spira, J., & Spiegel, D. (1993). Group psychotherapy for the medically ill. In A. Stoudemire & B. Fogel (Eds.), *Psychiatric care of the medical patient* (2nd ed., pp. 31–50). New York: Oxford University Press.

Stanton, A., & Reed, G. (2002). *The breast cancer notebook: The healing power of reflection.* Washington, DC: American Psychological Association.

Steggles, S., Maxwell, J., Lightfoot, N. E., Damore-Petingola, S., & Mayer, C. (1997). Hypnosis and cancer: An annotated bibliography 1985–1995. *American Journal of Clinical Hypnosis,* 39, 187–200.

Sullivan, H. S. (1953). *Interpersonal theory of psychiatry.* New York: Norton & Co.

Taylor, S. E., & Armor, D. A. (1996). Positive illusions and coping with adversity. *Journal of Personality,* 64, 873–898.

Telch, C. F., & Telch, M. J. (1986). Group coping skills instruction and supportive group therapy for cancer patients: A comparison of strategies. *Journal of Consulting and Clinical Psychology,* 54, 802–805.

Thoresen, C., & Bracke, P. (1997). Reducing coronary recurrences and coronary prone behavior: A structured group treatment approach. In J. Spira (Ed.), *Group psychotherapy for medially ill patients* (pp. 92–132). New York: Guilford Press.

Trijsburg, R. W., van Knippenberg, F. C. I., & Rijpma, S. E. (1992). Effects of psychological treatment on cancer patients: A critical review. *Psychosomatic Medicine,* 54, 489–517.

Watson, M., & Greer, S. (1998). Psychological and behavioral factors in cancer risk and survival: Personality and coping. In J. Holland (Ed.), *Textbook of psychooncology* (pp. 91–98). New York: Oxford University Press.

Watson, M., Greer, S., Pryun, J., & Van Den Borne (1990). Locus of control and mental adjustment to cancer. *Psychological Reports,* 66, 39–48.

Wellisch, D. K., Wolcott, D. L., Pasnau, R. O., Fawzy, F. I., & Landsverk, J. (1989). An evaluation of the psychosocial problems of the home-bound cancer patient: Relationship of patient adjustment to family problems. *Journal of Psychosocial Research,* 7, 55–76.

World Health Organization. (1996). *International classification of diseases* (10th ed.). Geneva: Author.

Yalom, I. D. (1980). *Existential psychotherapy.* New York: Basic Books.

Yalom, I. (1985). *Theory and practice of group psychotherapy* (3rd ed.). New York: Basic Books.

Yalom, V. J., Yalom, I. D. (1990). Brief interactive group psychotherapy. *Psychiatric Annals, 20*(17), 362–367.

Yuasa, N. (1966). *Basho: The narrow road.* New York: Penguin.

Zonderman, A. B., Costa, P., & McCrae, R. R. (1989). Depression as a risk for cancer morbidity and mortality in a nationally representative sample. *Journal of the American Medical Association, 262,* 1191–1195.

Author Index

Subject Index

About the Authors

James L. Spira, PhD, MPH, ABPP, is a licensed psychologist, board certified in clinical health psychology from the American Board of Professional Psychology. He received his doctorate in counseling psychology from the University of California at Berkeley and completed a postdoctoral fellowship at Stanford University School of Medicine emphasizing psychosocial oncology. Dr. Spira has served on the faculty of the Medical Schools at Duke University and the University of North Carolina at Chapel Hill and has been a consultant for numerous medical centers and organizations throughout the United States, Europe, and Australia over the past 15 years, helping establish psychosocial intervention programs for medically ill patients, particularly psychosocial oncology programs, and providing training for therapists. Dr. Spira has written several books, including *Group Therapy for Medically Ill Patients* and *Treating Dissociative Identity Disorder* and several therapist training manuals, as well as dozens of chapters and research articles. His current research focuses on the benefits of psychosocial interventions for medically ill patients for improved quality of life and psychophysiological processes. He serves on the Board of Directors for the American Board of Clinical Health Psychology and is on the editorial boards of several health psychology journals. Currently, Dr. Spira directs the Health Psychology Division at the

Naval Medical Center in San Diego, where he is also research coordinator for Mental Health Services and serves on the hospital's Committee for the Protection of Human Subjects. Dr. Spira is also a long-time student of Zen meditation and martial arts.

Geoffrey M. Reed, PhD, is a clinical and health psychologist. His clinical work and research has focused on responses to life-threatening illnesses, including AIDS and breast cancer, and he has published numerous scientific and policy articles in such journals as *American Psychologist, Health Psychology, Professional Psychology: Research and Practice*, and the *Journal of Social Issues*. While a member of the research faculty of the Department of Psychiatry and Biobehavioral Sciences at the University of California at Los Angeles, he was named one of the 50 Most Innovative AIDS Researchers in the US by *POZ Magazine*, a publication by and for people living with HIV. Dr. Reed is currently assistant executive director for professional development at the American Psychological Association (APA). In this position he is responsible for the development and implementation of collaborative marketplace demonstration projects focused on improving health care outcomes and patient care. He is a leading expert in the organization of health care systems, the measurement of health care processes and outcomes, and information infrastructure for health care systems and has consulted to a wide range of health care organizations. As a part of his work at APA, he has consulted to the U.S. Department of Defense on the integration and reorganization of the Army, Navy, and Air Force health care services in the National Capital Area. He has also worked extensively with the World Health Organization (WHO) on the implementation of WHO's International Classification of Functioning, Disability, and Health, a system designed to capture the functional consequences of health conditions. Most recently, he has been responsible for the design and implementation of a new Internet-based infrastructure for the collection of information regarding psychological practice.